Hypnosis
for a Joyful
Pregnancy and
Pain-Free Labor
and Delivery

Also by Winifred Conkling

The Expectant Mother's Checklist
Secrets of Echinacea
Secrets of Ginseng
Secrets of Gingko
The Carnitine Connection

Hypnosis

for a

Joyful Pregnancy

and

Pain-Free
Labor and Delivery

■ ■ ■

Winifred Conkling

Foreword by Nancy Barwick, D.C.H.

A Lynn Sonberg Book

 St. Martin's Griffin 〽 New York

www.stmartins.com

Library of Congress Cataloging-in-Publication Data

Conkling, Winifred.
    Hypnosis for a joyful pregnancy and pain-free labor and delivery—1st U.S. ed.
        p. cm.
    ISBN 0-312-27023-2
    1. Hypnotism in obstetrics—Popular works.   2. Natural childbirth—Popular works.   I. Title.
    RG661.C657
    618.4'5—dc21   2001041973

10 9 8 7 6 5 4 3 2

AUTHOR'S NOTE

This book is for informational purposes only. It is intended to tell you about methods of managing the discomfort associated with childbirth, but it should not take the place of medical advice from a trained medical professional. Readers are advised to consult an obstetrician or other qualified health-care professional before acting on any of the information in this book. The use of hypnosis for pain control should be carried out with the support of your obstetrician or other health-care provider.

The fact that an organization or Web site is listed in the book as a potential source of information does not mean that the author or publisher endorses any of the information it provides or recommendations it makes.

CONTENTS

FOREWORD

Birth is a universal human experience; it is the only way to begin a life. So why is the birth experience so different across cultures and times? Why, specifically, is it so closely associated with pain and danger in Western societies, when it can be accomplished in a hut without running water in less-affluent societies?

This seeming contradiction can be explained quite simply. In Western cultures, we have been taught that birth is a terrible ordeal. The truth of the matter, however, is quite different. Birthing can be a comfortable and even pleasant experience for the mother and baby. Relaxation, preparation, and information are the key ingredients, along with an understanding and a belief that birthing can be pain free.

Because our bodies and minds are intimately connected, mental activity and belief have an effect on the body. The person who delays a cold long enough to finish a project, the football player who plays despite injuries, the parent who stays awake throughout the night with a colicky baby are all able to do these things because the mind is in charge of the body. This is as it should be.

Mothers all over the world give birth every day in deep relaxation. Using their minds, these women relax their bodies so that their uteruses can do the work for which they were designed. The result is that the muscles work as they should and the babies are born more quickly, easily, and comfortably. Hypnosis and self-hypnosis are methods to achieve deep relaxation so that women can give birth to their babies naturally and comfortably. Birth can and ought to be easy for most mothers. The mothers with whom we work know that this is true; they experience it.

Hypnosis for a Joyful Pregnancy and Pain-Free Labor and Delivery is a wonderful book. It explains beautifully and cogently the story of birth and the process of hypnotherapy. The information is presented clearly and concisely so that all women can easily benefit from the techniques described here. As a hypnobirthing practitioner, I recommend this book to women and their partners who would like more information on birthing and relaxation.

NANCY BARWICK,
Doctor of Clinical Hypnotherapy,
Fairfax, Virginia

INTRODUCTION

Modern medicine offers a number of drugs that can be used to control the pain of childbirth, but each of them has the potential to cause harm to mother or baby or both. Of course, the vast majority of women who use anesthesia or pain medications during delivery experience no complications, but it is essential that women appreciate the possibilities of unwanted side effects. Fortunately, there is a 100 percent safe, natural alternative to drugs for pain control: hypnosis.

Hypnosis is the only form of anesthesia that presents no risk of complications to either mother or child. It is noninvasive and nontoxic, and it allows a woman to fully experience the joy of childbirth—without anxiety, fear, or labor pain. Kylie Mikuta, a twenty-six-year-old first-time mother, used hypnosis and experienced a pain-free delivery. "Women's bodies are made to give birth, and I didn't want my fear to get in the way of my birth experience," she said. "During delivery I was very calm. It was wonderful. I felt pressure, like menstrual cramps, but I can't say that I felt any pain. I kept expecting pain, but it never came. I was very surprised."

By the time Kylie's eight-pound, five-ounce daughter was born, she had been practicing hypnosis twice a day for about four months. "Everything that happened felt very natural," Kylie said. "When I was pushing, I was talking to my baby, asking her to come out, 'Come on out. I love you and I want to hold you.' It was the greatest experience of my life."

Unfortunately, Kylie's experience is relatively rare. Hypnosis is not widely used as a form of anesthesia in America today. Perhaps the major reason the technique is underutilized is that it is not fully understood by medical doctors. Even experts who have spent their careers researching hypnosis cannot completely explain exactly how it works.

People who have studied hypnosis generally agree that a hypnotic trance involves an altered state of awareness in which you concentrate so intensely that your subconscious mind becomes highly responsive to suggestion and able to tune out distractions. In this state of highly focused concentration, you can use the power of your mind to alter your perception of pain, including the pain generally associated with childbirth.

What Hypnosis Is and Isn't

Hypnosis as a method of pain control during labor and delivery is new to many women, but the technique has been used in surgery and in obstetrics since the 1820s. Hypnosis has fallen in and out of favor over the years, following the trends of medical practice. Currently American women are gaining a renewed appreciation of natural medicine and drug-free methods of healing, and there has been a corresponding increase in interest in hypnosis as anesthesia during childbirth.

As you learn more about hypnosis, you will find that it has much in common with many prepared childbirth techniques. Hypnosis, like these other methods, involves training in relaxation, anxiety reduction, deep breathing, and the use of imagery and psychological suggestion to cope with pain. But, unlike these methods, hypnosis allows you to enter a dream-like trance whenever you choose, and it works by communicating with the subconscious mind.

A hypnotic trance feels a lot like daydreaming. Your brain functions in a state of consciousness that involves the alpha brain-wave frequency, the same frequency used when you are daydreaming or fantasizing. During these times you are awake and fully aware of your surroundings, but you are able to screen out and disregard outside noises and other distractions.

At the most basic level, hypnosis involves training your mind to slip into this alpha wave state of super concentration. When you become proficient at hypnosis, you will be able to reach a state of acute relaxation and concentration within seconds. When your mind enters this state, it is highly responsive to suggestions, as long as what is being suggested is something you want to achieve. Hypnosis cannot be used to make you do anything you do not want to do, but it can be used to help you achieve goals you might not be able to attain without full concentration. With hypnosis you can learn to work with your subconscious and to achieve an anesthetic effect without the use of drugs or other potentially harmful approaches to pain control.

Many people think of hypnosis as a type of meditation, but there is an important distinction between the two practices. With meditation, your brain settles into alpha brainwave activity as you repeat a word or mantra. With hypnosis, you enter the alpha state, then you introduce suggestions with the explicit goal of changing your behavior, whether your goal is to control pain, break a two-pack-a-day smoking habit, or diminish your desire to snack on potato chips between meals.

Hypnosis has proved very successful for women preparing for childbirth because it allows them to get in touch with their natural ability to give birth. Modern obstetric practices tend to manage childbirth as a medical problem rather than to facilitate it as a natural bodily process. The contractions of labor begin spontaneously at the end of pregnancy, and they end with the delivery of a baby. In many cases, pregnant women are expected to be passive recipients of medical care during delivery, but this need not be the case. Hypnosis can be used to help a woman relax and work with her body during this completely natural process.

Using This Book

Hypnosis for a Joyful Pregnancy and Pain-Free Labor and Delivery can help you develop the hypnotic skills you need to enter a trancelike state and manage discomforts during labor and delivery. The pain of childbirth, like any other type of pain, is controlled by the brain. By teaching your mind and your body to accept and embrace the uterine contractions of childbirth, you can reinterpret and diffuse the sensation of this "pain."

The first chapter of the book describes the history of hypnosis and how it has been used for pain control in many settings. The second chapter outlines the biological process of childbirth and explains how hypnosis can be an effective form of anesthesia during labor and delivery. If you understand what is happening to your body during labor and delivery, you will realize that childbirth is nothing to fear. Rather than approaching your baby's birthday with anxiety, you can embrace the experience for the miracle that it is. Chapter 3 describes how you can determine whether you are a good candidate for hypnosis.

The rest of the book offers practical advice that can help you put hypnosis to work for you. Chapter 4 describes clearly the phases of a hypnotic trance and explains the purpose of each part of the session, from the induction to the closing. It provides an overview of hypnosis that will allow you to begin practicing the technique on your own, with a partner, or with a professional hypnotherapist, preferably one with experience dealing with pregnancy. Chapter 5 includes sample scripts for hypnosis, which can be read by a partner or tape-recorded and played at your convenience. Chapter 6 covers ways that hypnosis can be used to manage some of the common complaints of pregnancy, such as morning sickness and excess weight gain. Chapter 7 explains how you can find qualified hypnotherapists and other professionals to assist with your birth experience. Chapter 8 answers common questions about hypnosis.

Finally, Chapter 9 discusses common types of anesthesia. In some cases, medical intervention is necessary and anesthesia may be required. Your training in hypnosis may help you minimize your need for anesthesia, but there are situations when you may choose to use medication. If your labor and delivery do not go as you planned, do not see this as a failure or a sign of weakness on your part. Keep in mind that the ultimate goal of childbirth is a healthy baby and a healthy mother. In some cases, interventions and anesthesia are medically necessary. The hypnotic skills you learn will help you relax and minimize anxiety, no matter what kind of birth experience you have.

Hypnosis for a Joyful Pregnancy and Pain-Free Labor and Delivery

1

■ ■ ■   MESMERIZED
A Brief History of Hypnosis

For thousands of years, both men and women considered agonizing pain to be an inevitable part of childbirth. Suffering during labor and delivery was accepted as part of the price that all women must pay for original sin. Pain relief was considered a violation of God's will and a disruption of the natural order. In fact, women who attempted to use anesthesia or other means of pain relief were treated as heretics. For example, in 1591, a woman in Edinburgh, Scotland, requested pain relief while giving birth to twins. She was convicted of acts "contrary to divine law and in contempt of the Crown" and ultimately burned at the stake.

Fortunately, times have changed. Punitive suffering need not be part of modern childbirth. Virtually all midwives and health-care practitioners strive for relaxed, successful birth experiences, whether or not they use hypnosis with their patients. While the word *hypnosis* continues to conjure up images of entertainers who make willing subjects quack like ducks or perform other embarrassing acts, it is also used by thousands of medical doctors, midwives, psychiatrists, and psychologists.

Though the practice has not always been defined as hypnosis, the induction of a trance state is part of human nature. Mothers instinctively rock their babies back and forth and pat them on the back to sooth them and induce an almost hypnotic state of calm. Even though mothers have depended on such techniques to comfort their babies for eons, the actual practice of hypnosis was not formalized until about 250 years ago.

Meet Dr. Mesmer

Modern hypnotherapy started in the mid-eighteenth century when Viennese physician Friederich Anton Mesmer (1734–1815) set forth his theory of "animal magnetism." Mesmer hypothesized that the body contained a magnetic fluid that ebbed and flowed in accordance with an internal tide that responded to the tides of the oceans and the gravitational pull of the planets. He believed that illnesses were caused by imbalances of the body's tides and that a more harmonious distribution of magnetic fluid could cure disease. To patients afflicted with illness or disease, Mesmer offered a simple cure. He had them drink a potion that contained iron, and he created an "artificial" tide by attaching magnets to their bodies and transferring his fluid magnetism to them. This focus on magnets resulted in the term "animal magnetism."

Mesmer believed that the "magnetic fluid" could be transferred from one person to another, or, more precisely, from himself to his patients. Mesmer's healing rituals involved a dramatic display of hand waving and moving magnets in front of his patients while offering soothing words to calm them. He brought his patients into a state of focused attention; even today we say a person is "mesmerized" when he or she is entranced or in a state of deep concentration.

Mesmer's version of hypnosis became very popular for a time, but then his colleagues in Austria labeled him a charlatan. Still confident of his technique, Mesmer moved to Paris in the 1780s and was considered a miracle healer for a number of years. At the peak of his popularity, Mesmer held mass healings in which he filled large oak tubs with "magnetized" water, iron filings, and broken glass. As many as twenty people held metal rods that protruded from the sides of the tub. By touching the metal rods, people believed that the energy of the water flowed into their bodies and stimulated the circulation of the magnetic fluid within them.

While many people were impressed with Mesmer's abilities, others were less sure of them. One of the final straws came in 1784 when Mesmer suggested that women need not suffer pain during childbirth. That same year, a royal commission of Louis XVI, headed by Benjamin Franklin who was visiting overseas, determined that all that took place during one of Mesmer's healings was an "excitement of the imagination." Mesmer himself acknowledged that animal magnetism "must in the first place be transmitted through feeling." He recognized the importance of emotion in his healings, and he had an impressive, imposing air similar to that of a modern-day faith healer. He also was able to make pointed suggestions, often telling his patients in great detail what was going to happen to them. In essence, Mesmer's colleagues played down his success and attributed it to the placebo effect, in which a person's expectations trigger a response.

Refining the Practice of Hypnosis

Despite the scientific establishment's rejection of mesmerism, other healers were intrigued by the practice. One of the best known was a Hindu-Portuguese priest, Abbe José de Faria, who began to look at the practice in more analytical terms. In 1819 he concluded that the cause of the trance state (which he called "lucid sleep") was caused not by magnetism but by concentration by the subject. Faria had his clients relax, lean back, empty their minds, and concentrate on falling asleep, which most promptly did. He could then induce them to feel illusions of heat and cold and to experience various tastes and smells.

Faria had his patients stare at a stationary object, a hypnotic technique now called fixed-gaze hypnosis. He found that after his patients stared at the object and reached a point of heightened concentration, they were in a highly suggestible mood. At that point he commanded them to stop feeling their symptoms. In this way he produced near miraculous healings.

During this period, medical experts were gaining a greater appreciation for the mechanics of hypnosis. In the mid-nineteenth century, Dr. James Braid, a well-known surgeon from Manchester, England, coined the word *hypnosis*, after Hypnos, the Greek God of sleep. Rather than referring to what transpired in a trance as animal magnetism, he referred to it as "nervous sleep" brought on by hypnotic suggestion.

Braid was also the first to attribute the success of hypnosis to psychological rather than physical variables.

Like his colleagues, Braid had been very skeptical of mesmerism and animal magnetism, but he was intrigued with the practice after watching a mesmerist from France in 1841. Braid then began to experiment with hypnosis, and he eventually refined his technique, then used it to perform pain-free surgery after inducing a trance in the patient by staring at his subjects with a focused, authoritative gaze. Braid used hypnosis routinely in his medical practice during the 1840s and 1850s. He knew from experience that he was able to bring on a relaxed, sleeplike state in his patients, but he did not know why he was able to do so. Braid appreciated that the mind and body were intertwined, but he did not understand how the two interacted.

Another major breakthrough came when word spread of the work of Dr. James Esdaile, a British doctor working in India who used hypnosis as anesthesia when he performed as many as two thousand major operations, including at least nineteen amputations. Dr. Esdaile either passed his hands over the affected body part or simply pointed his finger at the patient until he or she entered a trance.

Hypnosis in the Twentieth Century

Hypnosis remained in vogue in some circles into the late nineteenth century. At that time, a respected French doctor, Dr. Hypolite Bernheim, founded the Nancy (France) School of Hypnotism. One of Dr. Bernheim's students was the well-known Viennese therapist Dr. Sigmund Freud who was intrigued by the practice of hypnosis. Freud used hypnosis to help patients explore how their feelings about past experiences might contribute to their current emotional problems. As his practice developed, Freud turned from hypnosis to other techniques, such as free association and dream interpretation, which became the cornerstones of psychoanalysis, but Freud readily acknowledged that many of his ideas about the human psyche began with his interest in hypnosis.

Medical practices tend to rise and fall in popularity, and psychoanalysis and other practices overshadowed hypnosis in the early part of the twentieth century. Hypnosis fell out of favor until the 1950s when Dr. Milton Erickson began experimenting with it for the treatment of both mental and physical ailments. Dr. Erickson is probably the best-known hypnotist of the twentieth century; his research on the practice has influenced thousand of hypnotists, psychotherapists, and hypnotherapists. Dr. Erickson's work demonstrated that hypnosis could be used to help people internalize new ways of thinking and behaving without being aware that they were learning.

Dr. Erickson's work legitimized hypnosis in the eyes of the medical community. In 1955, the British Medical Association approved hypnotherapy as a valid medical treatment and an effective form of pain control during childbirth. The association stated, "In suitable subjects, it [hypnosis] is an effective method of relieving pain in childbirth without altering the normal course of labour." The American Medical Association followed suit in 1958, concluding, "The use of hypnosis has a recognized place in the medical armamentarium and is a useful technique in the treatment of certain illnesses, when employed by qualified medical personnel."

Today, the therapy is so widely accepted that the American Society of Clinical Hypnosis, a professional association of physicians, psychologists, and dentists, boasts more than four thousand members. Hypnosis is now mainstream. It is even recognized by many health-maintenance organizations.

When it comes to the use of hypnosis in childbirth in the United States, no one has contributed more than Dr. Joseph B. DeLee, an obstetrician who took the radical stand of openly arguing that a woman need not suffer in childbirth. He realized in the 1930s, when hypnosis was out of vogue, that with hypnosis some women could relax profoundly during labor and delivery. Dr. DeLee advocated hypnosis as being the "only anesthetic without danger" and told the profession: "I am irked when I see my colleagues neglect to avail themselves of this harmless and potent remedy."

In the past fifty years, thousands of studies have validated the experience of Dr. DeLee and measured the efficacy of hypnosis. Today most people accept the mind-body connection and do not find it extraordinary to believe that the way a person thinks can alter the response of his or her body's systems, including the autonomic or involuntary body systems (such as temperature and blood pressure). Many modern health-care practitioners may find this result unremarkable, but at the time this was considered an unbelievable, incredible, and unexplainable claim.

Now you, too, can capture the power of the mind-body connection and use it for a more joyful, pain-free childbirth.

But first you have to practice the techniques outlined in this book, ideally with the help of a trained hypnotherapist. The next chapter will help explain the mechanics of childbirth and describe how hypnosis can be used as an alternative to anesthesia.

2

■ ■ ■ GREAT EXPECTATIONS
Childbirth Does Not Have to Be Painful

You already know a lot about giving birth, even if you haven't attended a single childbirth class or read a single page about labor and delivery. Childbirth is a natural process, although many treat it like a medical emergency. Women no longer rely on instinct and listen to their bodies to experience childbirth; instead, they approach labor with fear and anxiety and turn to doctors and anesthesiologists to orchestrate the process.

When thirty-two-year-old Sarah Rodgers entered the final stages of her pregnancy, her friends and family were surprised at her attitude about childbirth. "People told me that I should be scared and that if I wasn't frightened it was because I didn't know what I was talking about," she said. "Strangers told me stories about difficult births, but I remained calm. Childbirth just made sense to me; my body was designed to have a baby. The process is completely natural."

Sarah's confidence and calm demeanor, which were reinforced by regular sessions of hypnosis, helped her face childbirth with a positive attitude. She gave birth to her eight-pound, eight-ounce daughter in what she described as a pain-free delivery.

Most women don't have the confidence in their bodies that Sarah exemplifies. Instead, they have accepted the notion of agonizing labor portrayed in television sitcoms. As a result, they bring with them to the delivery room a significant amount of fear and insecurity. In many cases childbirth classes validate these feelings by presenting a picture of childbirth that involves fetal monitors, forceps, vacuum extractors, caesarean deliveries, and epidural anesthesia. All too often, what "prepared childbirth" classes prepare a woman for is a very medicalized and invasive birth experience.

In truth, the average woman is capable of giving birth without medications or interventions, as long as she is supported throughout her labor and trained to keep her mind focused by using a technique such as hypnosis. However, without an appreciation for the natural process of childbirth—and without confidence in their bodies—many women enter the delivery room in a state of terror, which only exacerbates their discomfort. This rapidly becomes a negatively reinforced cycle of fear and pain, which typically ends with a woman requesting (or begging for) anesthesia to control pain.

When we doubt ourselves and our ability to give birth, we also increase the chances that we will need medical interventions during the delivery. Of course, special circumstances can demand medical intervention, but most women have the potential to give birth naturally and without extraordinary measures.

Hypnosis helps a woman achieve her goal of natural childbirth by giving her an appreciation for what her body can do on its own. "Hypnosis is usually used by women who have had a baby and didn't like the experience, and by first-time mothers who are frightened," said Nancy Barwick, a hypnotherapist in Virginia who is trained in the hypnobirthing technique of hypnosis for childbirth. "Hypnosis gives women the confidence they need. It can make all the difference in the world in how a woman experiences childbirth."

Childbirth 101

Every pregnant woman needs to understand the mechanics of labor and delivery so that she can appreciate what is happening to her body during childbirth. Knowledge builds confidence and diminishes fear, allowing a woman to work with her body. The more you know, the less labor hurts, and the more effective hypnosis will be.

Even though every labor is different, in general, first babies take about twelve to fourteen hours of labor. Second and subsequent babies arrive after eight to ten hours of labor. However, as you know from hearing other mothers' birth stories, there is a wide range of experiences; some women are fast and give birth after five hours or less, and others can experience light labor for twenty-four hours or more.

In each of these labors, however, a woman's body goes through three very specific stages.

Stage 1: Opening of the Cervix

When your baby is ready to be born, he or she will let you know. For many women, labor starts with a feeling of discomfort or cramping in the lower back. It is followed by a tightening of the uterus, which makes the entire abdomen feel as hard as a basketball. Many women describe labor as severe menstrual cramps, which grow increasingly regular and rhythmic.

Most women experience some early irregularly spaced contractions on and off during the last month or so of pregnancy. These practice contractions help to get the uterus ready for the big day. They tend to be noticeable but mild.

Unlike these early contractions, the contractions of true labor are fairly evenly spaced. They may start out as much as twenty minutes apart, then become more frequent. They also build in intensity and duration as your body gets into its own rhythm.

Keep in mind that the purpose of labor is to allow your baby to pass through the expanding birth canal. The first step is to get the cervix, the neck of the uterus, to open wide enough to let the baby through. The uterine contractions gradually force open the cervix, but the process takes hours in most women.

The cervix is often described as similar in appearance to the opening of a turtleneck sweater. The neck of the sweater (the cervix) must open before you can push your baby down and out of the uterus. Most of labor is spent opening the cervix. In fact, if a woman has a textbook fourteen-hour labor, the only thing that happens for about twelve of those hours is that the cervix is opening. When the cervix is fully open (ten centimeters, or four inches), a woman's body has one long canal instead of a separate uterus and vagina. At this point, she is ready to push the baby out. So the real work of labor, the long work that takes most of time spent in labor, involves stretching open the neck of that turtleneck. This task, the opening of the cervix, is called the first stage of labor.

When the baby descends into the birth canal, the cervix is pulled open and back over the baby's head (just like a turtleneck). The cervix is drawn into the upper body of the uterus. When this occurs, the upper part of the uterus actually gets a little thicker, which helps it build strength to push the baby out.

So what pulls the cervix back and over the baby's head? Contractions. There is nothing particularly special about a uterine contraction. A muscle flexing or shortening is all a contraction is. And at the most basic level, that is all labor is: muscles involuntarily contracting and relaxing.

Some women dilate at a fairly even pace, perhaps about a centimeter an hour. Others measure four centimeters dilated one hour and then jump to ten centimeters the next. It is possible for a woman to get stuck at three or four centimeters for hours before opening farther; sometimes these transitions happen quickly. Even though it can be encouraging to see steady, measurable progress, knowing how far dilated you are really tells you nothing about how many more minutes or hours until you give birth. You must allow your body to prepare for delivery at its own pace. You can't hurry things along with sheer will.

You can, however, keep your labor on track by staying calm and comfortable. The more relaxed you are during labor, the easier and shorter your labor will be. A survey of some 1,000 women at a Chicago hospital found 306 cases in which labor began between midnight and 6 A.M., hours when the mothers were most likely to be resting. Only 182 women in the study started labor between the busier hours of noon and 6 P.M. Relaxation helps the body prepare for labor.

Hypnosis is very effective in the first stage of labor. With training and practice, you can use hypnosis to remain comfortable and free from fear or anxiety. The contractions may become more intense during "transition," the final part of stage 1, when the cervix is opening fully. If you experience any discomfort, your partner or doctor can help to induce a deeper hypnotic state and to reinforce the suggestion of relaxation.

"There is no pathological reason for pain in childbirth," said Marie Mongan, founder of the HypnoBirthing Institute in Pembroke, New Hampshire. "It's the fear that creates the tension and pain. Remove the tension and you can eliminate the pain."

About Contractions

Think of the uterus as three layers of muscle tissue. These muscles extend from the top of the uterus to the cervix. When these muscles contract, they shorten and flex, stretching and pulling open the cervix.

After flexing, the uterine muscles relax and gather strength. In early labor, a woman's muscles may flex for thirty seconds at a time then rest for five, ten, or even twenty minutes. Gradually, the uterus begins to flex for forty-five seconds at a time, followed by a rest of five minutes or less. A bit later, the uterine muscles may contract for sixty to seventy seconds and rest only two or three minutes between contractions. Finally, at the end of the first stage of labor, the uterus may flex for ninety seconds and rest for as little as one and a half to two minutes before flexing again.

These contractions help to pull the neck of the cervix flat against the baby's head. When this happens, the cervix is not opening, it is merely flattening out. Think of the turtleneck sweater pulled flat across your head but not yet pulled down over your head. This process of flattening is called effacement. During doctor visits in the last month of your pregnancy, your doctor may mention that your cervix is beginning to efface. If you're eager to deliver, you might get excited and think your baby's arrival is imminent. Calm down: Effacement tells you nothing at all about when labor will begin. You cannot predict when real labor will begin based on whether you have—or haven't—experienced any effacement.

Stage 2: Pushing

Once the cervix is open, it is time for the mother to push the baby out. The second stage of labor officially begins with her first push. Pushing can be tiring, but it can be exhilarating too, especially after a woman has learned how to work with her body.

During the second stage of labor, a woman still has contractions and rest periods, but now the contractions are known as pushing contractions. A woman's uterus is a powerful muscle that works almost like a piston to push the baby out. The uterine muscle applies about thirty-five to forty pounds of force, but the mother still needs to actively push to get the baby through the birth canal.

In this phase, most women experience rectal pressure, similar to the feeling associated with a bowel movement. This sensation is caused by the vagina enlarging as the baby moves through it and presses on the rectum. At this point a woman's obstetrician, midwife, or health-care provider will tell her when to draw in a deep breath, hold it, and push down throughout the contraction. Pushing comes very naturally; at that point, the body is focused on moving the baby through the birth canal and a woman instinctively knows when to push (unless she has had an epidural).

When a contraction ends, the baby may slip back a bit as the woman rests; this is perfectly natural. The uterus rests for a minute or two, then contracts again. This give and take typically continues for between a half hour and two hours, depending on the size of the baby, a woman's strength, and most important, whether this is a first vaginal delivery. Subsequent vaginal deliveries tend to go much faster because the tendons and muscles in the vagina have already been stretched by the previous birth.

Many women enjoy the sweaty, physically challenging but emotionally rewarding work involved in pushing during the second stage of labor. The second stage of labor officially ends when the baby is out.

After a woman has started pushing, but before the baby's head has emerged, some doctors perform a routine episiotomy, or a surgical incision along the perineum to give the baby more room to get out. This is similar to cutting the turtleneck to get it over your head without tearing the seams.

In most cases, the mother doesn't feel the cut because pressure from the baby's head cuts off the circulation to the perineum, making the area numb. After the baby is born, a local anesthetic may be injected into the perineum when the cut is being sutured or stitched because the area will have regained sensitivity since the baby has passed. (Some women do not want to undergo a routine episiotomy; discuss this matter with your obstetrician or health-care provider well in advance of your due date.)

The thought of your vagina expanding to the point that it can allow a full-term baby to pass though it may seem almost unbelievable, but keep in mind that your body has been preparing for this event throughout your pregnancy. Your body is meant to give birth; the mechanism for childbirth has been tested since the birth of man (literally) and it has proved to be quite effective. In addition, what you will experience is perfectly natural, and when you finally see your baby and listen to that first cry, you will be so overwhelmed with pride, satisfaction, wonder, and love that, despite your exhaustion, nothing else will matter.

Stage 3: Delivering the Placenta

The third stage is almost an afterthought. The work of childbirth is done, but the mother must push out the placenta or afterbirth. This usually happens spontaneously a few minutes after the baby is born.

It can be quite helpful to nurse your baby immediately after birth, if possible. Nursing at birth makes the uterus contract strongly and limits uterine bleeding. It also stimulates the production of oxytocin, a natural hormone that contracts the uterus and speeds the birth of the placenta. Once the baby is out, these final contractions cause the uterus to shrink.

That's it. Congratulations, Mom.

Wake Up, Baby

Although the birth process itself might sound a bit traumatic for the baby, this compression in the uterus and tight passage through the birth canal has a functional purpose. In addition to forcing the baby through the birth canal, uterine contractions stimulate the baby's entire body, readying its brain and nervous system for life outside the womb. In this brief transition from fetus to infant, a baby must make a number of radical adjustments. Outside of the mother's body, the baby must breathe, warm or cool himself or herself, regulate blood pressure, and eat by mouth—all for the first time.

Labor and the passage through the birth canal prepare babies for their life outside the womb in a way that nothing else can duplicate. The physical realities of labor stimulate the baby's adrenal glands to produce the hormones that allow the baby's body to function on its own. If a woman has a caesarean delivery, the baby is pulled out of the body through a surgical incision in the uterus and the baby does not experience the physical challenges of labor. Because they don't go through the squeezing and pushing involved in a vaginal delivery, caesarean-born infants are more likely to have initial problems clearing their lungs and getting breathing established. For the baby as well as the mother, birth can be exhausting, but it serves a vital function. During the first journey of its life, a child is not meant to be helpless or passive. It is meant to be awake and aware, a fully active participant.

Nothing to Fear

It is normal to experience fear when you encounter the unknown, especially when you encounter a physically challenging event such as childbirth. In all cultures, women tend to experience some fear or anxiety about childbirth, but modern Western women fear childbirth much more than women in other cultures and women in the past. The irony is that modern childbirth is safer and more successful than ever before.

Some experts believe that women's attitudes about their bodies and about childbirth have been so shaped by the medical profession that the birth experience they expect is nothing like the experience would be in a less institutionalized setting. In the past, women did not expect to go through life—and give life—without experiencing any discomfort. Today, our society tends to believe that life should be virtually pain free and that any situations that could involve discomfort should be managed with painkillers or medical intervention.

Fortunately, there is a growing movement today to get women back in touch with their natural childbearing abilities. Hypnosis is a tool that can help women overcome their fear of childbirth. When a woman is trained in hypnosis and takes the time for regular practice, she can recapture her childbearing instincts and approach childbirth without fear or pain.

Fear of pain in childbirth often becomes a self-fulfilling

prophesy. Fear causes tension, which in turn causes pain. Fear causes a tightening deep in the gut, shallow breathing or holding of breath, constriction in the throat, and tension in the muscles of the face, hands, arms, buttocks, and legs. The blood drains from the digestive system and to the muscles; we become pale, tense, and ready to flee.

This fear is misplaced, especially in modern childbirth. Today, doctors have the medical expertise and technology to solve most of the serious problems that can occur. Women need reassurance, not that medical science can help deliver a healthy baby, but that Mother Nature has already given them most of the tools they need to deliver a healthy baby on their own.

In primitive societies, women entered a trancelike state during labor by singing, chanting, or repeating prayers to take their mind off the pain of contractions or to change their state of consciousness so that the pain became only one element of the experience. Often, women today do the opposite: They focus so much of their attention on the pain—from early in pregnancy and birth classes right into labor—that they end up priming themselves for unendurable pain. In other words, women who anticipate pain experience pain. It is possible to prevent fear by using hypnosis and the power of the mind to shift the mind into a relaxed and tranquil state, even during the height of labor.

Haven't Got Time for the Pain

Pain is not all in your mind, but your mind does affect your perception of pain. Research done in World War II confirms this. During the war, Dr. Henry K. Beecher of Harvard University compared how two groups of men reacted to pain. One group of men were soldiers wounded on the battlefield in Italy; the others were American men hospitalized for various surgeries. The men injured in war reported relatively little pain from their injuries. Only about 25 percent of the badly wounded soldiers complained of enough pain to request medication seven to twelve hours after being injured, whereas more than 80 percent of the civilian men asked for painkillers after surgery. Dr. Beecher concluded:

> In a situation in which a wound has great advantage, and means escape from overpowering anxiety and fear of death on the battlefield (as in the case of war wounds terminating military service), extensive wounds are associated with comparatively little pain. In a situation in which the wound connotes disaster (for example, major surgery in civilian life), lesser wounds are associated with far more pain than in the former situation. The essential difference appears to be in the difference in anxiety level in the two cases, in the attitude of the patient, and in his reaction to his wound.

This research has helped us learn about differences in the perception of pain. When it comes to childbirth, obstetricians have long been aware that some women tolerate pain much better than others. One of the most significant factors determining how much pain a woman experiences is her level of fear.

Fear and anxiety trigger the body's "fight or flight" response, an instinctive reaction that prepares the body to handle a perceived threat by running away or doing battle. When under stress, a woman's uterus contracts and the cervix tightens. The greater the fear, the more intense the muscular reaction, and the harder the uterus must work to force the cervix open during labor. This situation can create the self-reinforcing cycle of fear, tension, and pain that can make even an uncomplicated birth experience difficult.

This fear-tension-pain cycle can be broken at any point. Medicinal anesthesia breaks the cycle at the point of pain; hypnosis breaks the cycle at the fear-tension point, before the body experiences pain. Hypnosis can help you relax and accept your contractions, minimizing tension in the body and allowing the birthing muscles to work in harmony.

The experience of thousands of women who have used hypnosis during childbirth has proved that hypnosis offers significant benefits, but researchers do not fully understand the biochemistry of what happens during hypnosis and childbirth. Some researchers believe that hypnosis encourages the natural release of mood-enhancing chemicals called enkephalins and endorphins that change the way the body perceives pain. Other researchers believe, in technical terms, that hypnosis somehow causes the frontal limbic system of the brain, which regulates body functions, to inhibit pain impulses from the thalamus (the sensory relay center of the brain) to the cortex (the part of the brain that handles the perception of sensory information). In other words, hypnosis actually alters the way the brain experiences pain, allowing childbirth to unfold without pain.

Whatever mechanism is at work, experts agree that in the

relaxed state of hypnosis, a woman is receptive to suggestions to ignore pain and to minimize muscular tension. Under hypnosis, a woman does not function like an unfeeling zombie. Instead, she experiences the sensations of labor and delivery, but she does not interpret them as pain. Even in the deepest state of hypnosis, a woman can feel her uterus contracting during labor, but she does not feel the contraction as pain. Instead, she may interpret the feeling as pressure or tightening, but without discomfort or unpleasantness.

It also needs to be mentioned that pain is not the enemy. Pain helps to protect the body from injury and disease. It is a warning system that tells us to pay attention to our bodies. In pregnancy, pain can indicate a problem that demands medical attention. For example, persistent headaches during pregnancy, especially in the third trimester, can indicate toxemia, a condition in which the blood pressure rises. This condition should be brought to your doctor's attention. You can use hypnosis to manage the natural process of labor and delivery, but discuss other complaints with your obstetrician or health-care provider.

The Mind-Body Connection

Every thought you have affects your body. Your emotions trigger physical reactions every day, whether you are pregnant or not. For example, worry can trigger digestive problems, such as ulcers and diarrhea; anger stimulates the adrenal glands, raising blood pressure and causing muscle tension. Anxiety stimulates blood flow, resulting in a rapid pulse rate and high blood pressure. These physical changes can be brought on by both conscious and subconscious thoughts. In the same way, they can be controlled by both conscious and subconscious suggestions.

Hypnosis takes advantage of this mind-body link. It helps to reprogram the subconscious by replacing old thinking with new thinking. Many women have internalized a message that childbirth is painful and unpleasant; hypnosis can help you internalize the concept that childbirth is rewarding, satisfying, and free of pain.

Using hypnosis to control pain in childbirth can benefit all pregnant women, including those who are planning to use epidural anesthesia during delivery. For one thing, childbirth doesn't always follow a given woman's plans or expectations; complications do arise. Every childbirth experience is different, so even a mother of other children may not know what to expect during delivery. Sometimes an anesthesiologist isn't available when you want an epidural, other times labor progresses so quickly that there is not time for one. In any case, you won't regret learning the techniques necessary to control pain using hypnosis.

Of course, you can't be certain that hypnosis will be entirely effective during your labor. Regular practice increases the odds that the technique will work because it gives your subconscious plenty of time to internalize the suggestions discussed later in this book. By practicing hypnosis, you prepare your mind for delivery, so that when the big moment arrives, your subconscious mind is ready to help you have a rewarding childbirth experience.

Can You Relax Around Your Doctor?

If you plan to use hypnosis as anesthesia during childbirth, discuss this with your doctor as early as possible. Your doctor may have helpful suggestions about how to make the approach more successful, or may be able to recommend a professional who can help you with your training.

Don't stay with a doctor if you're not satisfied with his or her attitude toward hypnosis. Many women hesitate to switch doctors because they are afraid of insulting the physician or hurting his feelings. Your doctor won't remember the details of your birth one year from now, but you will remember the experience all of your life.

Most important, if you have anxiety about working with your doctor, or if you don't trust him or her fully, you will carry fear and tension with you into labor and it will be difficult to remain tranquil. Keep your birth experience your own. Circumstances you may not be able to foresee may alter your birth plan, but you can choose a doctor who shares your vision of the ideal birth.

3

■ ■ ■ ■ "YOU ARE FEELING
SLEEPY"
Are You a Good Candidate for Hypnosis?

Before investing a lot of time and energy in a program of hypnosis, you may want some assurance that the technique will be successful for you. Experts estimate that about 15 to 20 percent of the population is highly susceptible to hypnosis, about 15 to 20 percent is resistant to it, and everyone else falls somewhere in between. As a general rule, good candidates for hypnosis tend to be those who enjoy solitary activities, who can become absorbed in a project for long periods of time, who don't have difficulty trusting others, who prefer emotional to rational thinking, who tend to empathize with others, and who have vivid imaginations.

While there is no definitive test of susceptibility for hypnosis, the following tests may help to give you some idea of how easy it will be for you to enter a trance state. In fact, researchers who study hypnosis often use variations of these tests to determine which people will be good candidates.

To test yourself, you need the assistance of a partner or spouse who makes certain suggestions and monitors your behavior. These tests can give you a fairly good indication if you are easily hypnotized, but do not give up on the technique if you find any of them difficult or if you fail to respond. You may simply need to work with a professional who is better able to customize an approach that works for you.

Another benefit to taking time to perform these simple self-tests is that you will learn to respect the power of your imagination. Most people underestimate the power of their minds. You cannot achieve what you cannot imagine. When it comes to childbirth, you can learn to use the power of your mind to achieve the kind of birth experience that you desire.

- **The Whites of Your Eyes Test.** Sit in a chair facing your partner. Take a deep breath and relax. Open your eyes as wide as you can. Without tipping your head back, roll your eyes up into your head as far as you can. Look up at your eyebrows, your forehead, higher. . . . Keep your eyes skyward and lower your eyelids without allowing your eyes to come down. Have your partner look at the whites of your eyes. As a general rule, the greater the white area of your eyes that is exposed, the more susceptible you will be to hypnosis. Researchers cannot explain this phenomenon, but it is widely accepted as a screening test.

- **The Moving Light Test.** Sit comfortably in a darkened room. Have your partner stand across the room, holding a small flashlight. Your partner should move the light back and forth slightly, then ask, "Do you see the light moving?" He should then hold the light in a stationary position and again ask, "Do you see the light moving?" Most people will "see" the light move, even when it is in a fixed position; they tend to be good subjects for hypnosis.

- **The Lemon Test.** Sit comfortably and ask your partner to read the following script to you:

  > Close your eyes and take a deep breath. Exhale slowly. Imagine that you see a plump, yellow lemon on a table. Reach down and pick it up. Now hold it up to your nose and breathe in its citrus fragrance. Put it on the table and slice the lemon in half. See the juice drip out onto the table. Lift half the lemon and squeeze it into a glass. Watch the juice drip from the pulp. Raise the glass and take a sip, allowing the tart, citrus juice to wash over your tongue.

  Are you salivating? Many people actually pucker and salivate when they focus on the mental image of tasting a lemon. As you might expect, the better you are at responding to the visual image, the more likely you are to respond to hypnotic suggestions.

- **The Bucket of Water Test.** Sit comfortably in a chair and close your eyes. Ask your partner to read the following script to you:

  > Take a deep breath in. Now exhale. Sit squarely in your chair and extend both of your arms straight out. That's right. Now keep the palms of your hands facing the floor. Okay. Very good.
  > Now I would like you to close your eyes and imagine that I am placing two plastic buckets in

your hands. They are empty. They weigh almost nothing. Even with your eyes closed, you can see two buckets, one in each hand. Take a deep breath. As you breathe in, you will see the buckets more clearly. As you exhale, you will see them more clearly still.

You will remain relaxed as I slowly pour water from a glass pitcher into one of the buckets. You can choose which bucket I will pour into. Good choice. I have poured about one cup of water now, so the bucket is just a little bit heavier.

I am adding more water now. As you breathe in, you can feel me adding more water to the bucket. You can hear it splashing as it flows into the bucket. The bucket is filling with water and it is growing heavier. It is pulling your hand downward. The water is flowing into the bucket. It is heavier, heavier . . . heavier.

Keep your eyes closed and your arms out straight. Imagine the bucket, almost filled to overflowing. It is getting harder and harder to keep your arm up. Feel the bucket. Feel it pulling against your arm. Pulling down, down. Open your eyes.

Are your arms even? Is the arm holding the bucket filled with water higher than the other one? Your arms may be at different levels because you accepted the suggestion or because you were working hard to resist the suggestion you were being given. Either way, if your hands are not even, you used your imagination and your concentration to change your perception of your body. The more easily you responded to the mental image of holding the bucket of water, the more likely you will respond to hypnosis.

- **The Pendulum Test.** You can do this test on your own or with a partner. You will need a string or ribbon about fifteen inches long, a washer or a ring as a weight, and a piece of paper and pen.

  Tie the washer or ring at the end of the string or ribbon. On the paper, draw a circle and mark it north, south, east, west. Sit comfortably and rest your elbow on a table and hold the string between your thumb and index finger. Position your arm so that the weight falls right at the center of the circle. Ideally, your arm should be at a 45-degree angle to the table.

  Close your eyes and lift the pendulum about a quarter inch off the table. Take a deep breath and relax. Close your eyes and begin to think of the north-south direction. Try to hold your arm as still as possible. Think of the direction of the north-south line. Concentrate on the north-south axis.

  Open your eyes. In what direction is the pendulum swinging? Most people find that the pendulum swings in the direction of their thoughts. Without being aware of your motion, you may move your hand ever so slightly in response to your thoughts. You can experiment with east-west movements and with clockwise and counterclockwise rotations.

What Do You See
When You Close Your Eyes?

Are you a visual person, or do you find it difficult to "see" something using just your imagination? It's easy to find out with this self-test.

Close your eyes and think of a table, any table. When you have it in your mind, look it over and then open your eyes.

Did you actually "see" the table? What color was it? Was it wood or metal, plastic or some other material? What shape was it? When asked to perform this exercise, a visual person actually sees a particular table. A nonvisual person, on the other hand, knows what a table is and has a firm intellectual grasp of what a table looks like, but does not necessarily see a table. Interestingly, people who are not visual can understand what it would be like to process information visually, but people who are visual find it almost impossible to understand how someone can imagine something without "seeing" it. If this concept is difficult for you to grasp, you're probably a visual person.

If you "saw" a table, you can process information visually. If you did not, you may want to try nonvisual cues when customizing hypnotic suggestions. In other words, rather than using "see" the table or "visualize" the table, use "imagine" the table.

Putting Hypnosis to the Test

As you learn more about hypnosis and begin to work through the exercises in this book, you may still have some reservations about whether the technique is actually working. Specifically, you may experience that relaxation and hypnotic suggestions work well when resting comfortably on the couch but may fear that they will be less effective when contractions start hard and fast.

You can build your confidence—and learn more about which types of exercises will help you best manage your discomfort—by trying the following experiment.

Lie down on your left side on a comfortable couch or bed. Ask your partner to pinch you as tightly as he can on the flesh behind your knee. The pinch should last a full sixty seconds. The pressure should intensify during the first thirty seconds, reach a maximum intensity for ten seconds, then gradually decrease. The partner can explain that the "contraction" is coming, that the intensity of the squeeze is building, and that it will be over soon. This squeeze is intended to simulate a uterine contraction during labor. Rest for sixty seconds, then repeat the pinch.

Without using hypnosis, you will feel pain, a lot of pain. (If it doesn't hurt, your partner isn't pinching hard enough.) You also will learn about how you instinctively respond to pain.

Did you hold your breath? Did you breathe harder? Did you make noise as you exhaled deeply? Did you listen to your partner's voice? Did you talk to yourself (silently or aloud)? These are *auditory responses*.

Did you clench your fists, kick your feet, or bite your lip? Did you long for a hot or cold towel? These are *kinesthetic responses*.

Did you use visual imagery to put yourself somewhere else?

Did you imagine that you were on a beach or hiking in the mountains? Did you imagine your baby's face, or the images of other children? These are *visual responses*.

This exercise will help you determine if you tend to be auditory, kinesthetic, or visual in your coping mechanisms. This can be helpful as you design your hypnosis program and choose hypnotic suggestions that focus on your individual coping strategies. Sample hypnotic scripts are provided in Chapter 5, but the most effective are those you write yourself based on your experiences and your individual coping style.

One caveat: Do not hold your breath, even if this is an instinctive response for you. You must breathe through all of your contractions, to help you remain relaxed and ensure that both you and your baby receive all the oxygen you need. Your partner can remind you to relax and breathe deeply as a regular part of your hypnotic suggestion.

You should experiment with all types of coping mechanisms, but some will prove to be more effective for you than others. When using visual imagery, keep in mind that the images tend to be most effective when they match the pattern of your contractions. For example, when thinking of your cervix opening, you can focus on an image of a flower gradually opening its petals. Or when experiencing a wave of muscle contractions, you can imagine ocean waves washing up on the shore. The waves can come crashing down during the peak phase of a contraction, then ease as the contraction weakens. When the mind and body are in sync, this technique can be very effective.

You can use the pinch test both before and after you learn about hypnosis. Before working with hypnosis, the test can show you how you instinctively handle pain. Later, as you master the techniques of hypnosis, you can repeat it to demonstrate how effective the technique can be in helping you manage pain.

The various self-tests described in this chapter can help you build confidence in your hypnotic abilities, but the best way to determine your "talent" as a hypnotic subject is to give the technique a try. Keep in mind that the more you practice, the better you will be able to use hypnosis to unlock the power of your mind. Ultimately, with regular practice and concentration, you will be able to use your mind to help you fulfill your vision of the ideal childbirth.

4

■ ■ ■ SPECIAL DELIVERY

Using Hypnosis to Prepare for Delivery

Have you ever had a day when virtually everyone you meet stops and asks, "Are you feeling all right? You don't look well." Even if you felt quite chipper when you left the house in the morning, by the third or fourth time you are questioned about your health, you may wonder, "Why does everyone think I look sick? I guess I do look a little pale. I'm not really feeling so well. Maybe I'm getting a cold."

If you weren't sick before, you probably will be by the end of the day. No matter how healthy we are, the power of suggestion can be so great an influence that we can be made to believe that we are sick even if there is no physical cause for illness. It has also been shown that the mind's effect is so powerful on the body that many times we will, in fact, develop many of the symptoms of the disease or condition we believe we are catching. This you-are-what-you-think condition is not the exclusive right of psychosomatics and fakers. The power of the subconscious mind affects us all.

When used to your advantage, this phenomenon of suggestibility can be a very effective tool to reach your personal goals, whether they are to lose ten pounds, give up smoking, or experience a pain-free pregnancy.

Simply put, hypnosis is the process of using suggestibility to achieve our goals. We have all been hypnotized thousands of times without knowing it. When the ocean waves lull us into a dreamlike state of mind, when staring at the monotonous white line down the center of the highway causes our eyes to feel heavy, or when we get so wrapped up in a novel or movie that we lose track of time and cannot hear the sounds around us—these are all situations that involve the induction of a trancelike, hypnotic state.

Some people describe a hypnotic trance as similar to the dreamlike state you experience on mornings you hit the snooze button again and again. You know you're lying in bed, not quite asleep and not quite awake. In this midpoint between sleeping and waking, the subconscious rules.

During hypnosis the mind is focused to the point that it screens out ideas and stimuli in the world around us. When listening acutely to a piece of music, do you ever close your eyes to hear better? You instinctively do this to focus on what you are hearing; you may look like you are going to sleep, but you are actually more alert than you would be if you were doing more than one thing at once.

Many people inaccurately believe that being in a hypnotic trance is like being asleep. Just as you are more alert when listening intently, you are more alert when listening in a trancelike state. In fact, hypnosis is nothing more than a relaxed, highly focused state of attention. In a trance, you experience feelings of well-being, muscle relaxation, increased pain tolerance, diminished ability to vocalize, and an ability to accept new ideas about yourself if they are stated properly and not in conflict with your personal value system. Hypnosis involves guided imagery that helps your subconscious mind accept and internalize a specific goal.

In a hypnotic trance, you can hear and see everything that is going on around you. If, for example, a fire should break out, you would know to get up and leave the building just as rapidly as you would in a normal state of awareness. At every point of the process, you choose to continue in the trance; a person remains in a hypnotic trance because she has confidence in the process and believes the established goal is in her personal best interest.

For hypnosis to be successful, you must believe in the process and your goal. Your attitude about hypnosis—your faith, confidence, and expectations—determines how suggestible you are and how well the technique will work for you. If you believe in the power of hypnosis, it will work for you.

Hypnosis and Brain Waves

Researchers can measure the frequency of brain cycles. Not surprisingly, the speed of these cycles corresponds to different types of brain activity.

When you are in a hypnotic trance, your brain waves slow down and resemble those of sleep. Your thinking, conscious mind is quiet, and your subconscious mind is open.

As you fall asleep, your brain automatically slows down from the beta range into alpha and then for brief periods into theta and delta. Most of the time you sleep, your brain is in the alpha range. Hypnosis feels a bit like sleep because the brain slows down into the alpha range, allowing the subsconscious mind to open for suggestive input.

Experts agree on the types of brain waves and their general purpose, but they disagree on the exact boundaries of each kind of wave. The following is a basic consensus of the definitions of the four main types of brain waves.

- Delta: The frequency of brain activity ranges from zero to about four cycles per second. This is total unconsciousness. Not much is known about the delta range.

- Theta: The frequency ranges from about four to seven cycles per second. Theta is part of the subconscious range, and deeper stages of hypnosis can take place here. People tend to experience theta cycles in those moments when they are just falling asleep or awakening.

- Alpha: The frequency range is about seven to fourteen cycles per second. Alpha is usually regarded as the subconscious range. This is where dreaming (while asleep), daydreaming, meditation (though the brain waves can dip into theta during meditation), and most hypnosis take place. When you enter a light state of alpha activity, you have an increased awareness of anything perceived through the senses. We can enter the alpha range while listening to music or a sermon, reading a book, painting, daydreaming, driving, or doing any activity that requires focused attention.

- Beta: The frequency range is about fourteen cycles per second and higher. Beta involves the conscious, reasoning mind, where we operate most of the day.

Stages of Hypnosis

Although almost anyone can be hypnotized, not everyone can reach the deepest levels of hypnosis. With practice, you can become more proficient at hypnosis; most people can reach a deep enough state of hypnosis to experience anesthesia if they work at it.

Researchers recognize four major levels or depths of hypnosis.

- Light or "hypnoidal" state: This is characterized by deep physical relaxation, fluttering eyelids, and closed eyes.

- Cataleptic state: This is marked by catalepsy (or muscular rigidity) of the limbs, as well as the ability to reach anesthesia. When the muscles are cataleptic, they become up to 25 percent more efficient. Researchers have demonstrated this phenomenon by giving their subjects the suggestion to raise their arms as they feel themselves going deeper and deeper into a state of relaxation. When subjects reach the cataleptic state of hypnosis, their muscle strength is so great that it can be difficult for another person to bend the subjects' arms. In addition, the hypnotized person can keep an arm extended for an extraordinarily long period of time without tiring. While this is interesting, the more important thing that occurs in this stage is that a person can learn how to experience hypnotic anesthesia. The deeper the hypnotic trance, the more pain the body can ignore.

- Medium hypnosis: This state is characterized by partial amnesia, anesthesia, desirable personality changes, susceptibility to simple posthypnotic suggestions, and delusions of heat, cold, etc.

- Deep or somnambulistic state: This deepest state of hypnosis involves the ability to open your eyes without coming out of the trance, to respond to more complex hypnotic suggestions, to filter out or not hear distracting sounds, and to not see distracting images.

When you are hypnotized, you do not need to worry about what stage you are experiencing. You will not be aware of moving from one stage to another, though an experienced hypnotherapist may be able to distinguish when you reach a deeper state and are ready to accept more complex hypnotic suggestions. Keep in mind that the deeper the hypnosis, the more intense the susceptibility to suggestion. Hypnosis works on a continuum, and you can benefit from suggestions made at any point, though the deeper the trance, the more profound the changes and the greater your ability to withstand labor pains.

Getting Started

The time you spend learning hypnosis will pay off on your baby's birthday. Now that you appreciate the many advantages to using hypnosis for relaxation during labor, it's time to learn how to put the technique into practice. This chapter will help you better understand how you can enter a hypnotic trance and how you can frame positive suggestions that will help you minimize your perception of discomfort during your baby's birth. Chapter 5 provides sample scripts that you can use when experimenting with hypnosis at home.

Training in hypnosis usually begins in the sixth month of pregnancy, but it's never too early or too late to start. The more you practice, the better your skills, so make a commitment to practice regularly, no matter when you begin your training.

Early training allows you plenty of time to develop trust in your hypnotist and confidence in your own hypnotic ability. It also gives you time to experiment with various types of induction and visualization to find the approach that feels right for you.

You can work with hypnosis on your own, using this book and self-hypnosis audio- and videotapes, or you may want to work with a professional hypnotherapist. (For more information on finding a hypnotherapist, see Chapter 7.)

Before you get started, you need to open your mind to the possibilities of hypnosis. Forget all the images you have seen on television or in the movies and ignore the smug remarks from friends and family members who don't support your decision to try hypnosis. The more open-minded and accepting you are, the more likely this approach will work for you.

Along these same lines, it is essential to have faith in yourself and your ability to be hypnotized. If you believe you will be hypnotized, you will be. If you are ready to focus and follow your partner's suggestions, you will find it very easy and natural to reach your goals. If you focus on your hypnotherapist's words, you will find it almost impossible not to be hypnotized.

Setting the Scene

At the beginning of a hypnotherapy session, you want to create an environment that will allow you to focus without distraction. Keep the following tips in mind:

- Remove any jewelry, belts, or other accessories that may distract you.

- If you wear glasses, take them off.

- Do not chew gum or hard candies during your session.

- Loosen any tight clothing.

- You can either sit or lie down. Most people prefer to sit so that they don't feel sleepy.

- Take a trip to the bathroom before you get started. (This will become increasingly important during the third trimester as the baby grows and presses on your bladder.)

- If you are at home, take the phone off the hook or turn the ringer off.

- If you have other children, ask your spouse or a friend to watch them so you won't be interrupted.

Take a Deep Breath

Just before you begin your hypnosis session, take a deep breath. The way you breathe reveals a lot about how you are feeling. If you are tense or frightened, your breathing will be rapid and shallow. If you are relaxed and comfortable, your breathing will be deep and even. If you draw a deep breath, you will automatically begin to feel yourself relax.

If you watch a newborn breathe, you will see the abdomen raise and lower with each breath. The chest is still and the shoulders are relaxed. This is natural, deep breathing. Most adults have forgotten how to breathe deeply and instead draw shallow breaths into the upper part of the chest rather than the abdomen. This shallow breathing uses only about one-third of the lungs' capacity, allowing the fresh air to mix with the stale air, decreasing the body's supply of oxygen.

During labor, it is important that your breathing be calm, steady, and regular. You need to pay attention to your breathing so that you can keep an even rhythm during labor. Relaxed breathing causes the entire body to relax; you cannot feel panicky and out of control while practicing steady, deep breathing.

Take a deep breath. Do it again. Now you are ready to begin.

Induction: Slipping into a Trance

Whether you are working with a professional hypnotherapist, following the information in this book, or working with your spouse, you will use an induction to enter a hypnotic trance. There is nothing magical about this process; it is simply a way of focusing your attention.

There are a number of different types of inductions, but some of the most common involve watching a moving object go back and forth, staring at an imaginary spot on the ceiling directly above your forehead, or counting backward slowly from thirty, all while the hypnotherapist is using a monotonous, soothing voice to suggest that your eyes are getting heavy. (Sample scripts used for inductions are provided in Chapter 5.)

During the induction, you feel very relaxed. Your conscious mind fades, and you no longer feel the need to control every thought you have. Instead, you allow your partner's voice to lead you into a series of imaginative states. In this process, your surroundings become less important and your emotions become more important. You focus exclusively on the hypnotherapist's voice and suggestions.

At this point, you have entered a light state of hypnosis. You feel very relaxed, and you may feel more receptive to the hypnotherapist's suggestions. You may feel as if you are standing outside yourself, observing yourself in an unhurried, relaxed way. You feel very aware of your body and find it easy to focus on sensations you take for granted during the hustle of everyday life. For example, if your hypnotherapist suggests that you focus on the sensations in the ends of your fingertips, you are able to do so. The induction helps you settle down and prepare to enter a deeper hypnotic trance.

Deeper, Deeper, Deeper

The next phase of hypnosis involves deepening the feelings of relaxation. The more focused your concentration and the more relaxed you are, the more readily your subconscious accepts hypnotic suggestions. As you focus your attention, you find it easy to become more deeply hypnotized because other noises and distractions fade into the background.

The depth of your state of relaxation depends, in part, on the amount of trust you have in your hypnotherapist. Some people can slip right into the deepest stages of hypnosis in the first session, but for most people it takes longer. The more you practice, the more adept you will become at going into deeper and deeper hypnotic trances. (Sample scripts for deepening a trance are provided in Chapter 5.)

The Heart of the Matter: Hypnotic Suggestions

Once you experience the profound state of relaxation associated with hypnosis, your subconscious will accept suggestions. For pain relief during pregnancy, the suggestions involve ways to visualize or manage the discomfort so that it does not interfere with the enjoyment of your delivery.

When it comes to creating hypnotic suggestions, the possibilities are endless. (Some suggestions for language are included in Chapter 5.) However, you must choose your words with care, since the content of the message is critical to success. For hypnosis to be most effective, the suggestions should have a number of features.

- **Use positive suggestions.** Do not use the word *not*. State your goal using positive language. Also avoid saying *try*. (*Try* is a wishy-washy word; tell your subconscious you *will* achieve your goal, not just try to achieve your goal.) Do not use the word *pain;* instead mention *discomfort, pressure,* or *signal.*

  NO: I will not eat chocolate.

  YES: I am free of the desire to eat chocolate.

  NO: I will try not to yell at my children.

  YES: I am relaxed and loving when I speak to my children.

  NO: I will not experience pain during labor.

  YES: I feel gentle pressure on my cervix during labor.

- **State hypnotic suggestions in the present tense.** The subconscious likes to procrastinate. The changes you are making take effect right now, not in the future, so make your suggestions in the present tense.

  NO: I will not be afraid of childbirth.

YES: I enjoy giving birth to my baby.

NOTE: Some hypnosis scripts include the future tense—
you will . . . —because this statement helps make the
subconscious more receptive to a certain idea. In most
cases, the future tense is followed by a present-tense suggestion. In other words, a hypnotic script may include
language such as the following: "When I count to three,
you will feel relaxed. One . . . you feel relaxed . . ." and
so forth.

- **Choose specific words.** You are talking to your subconscious, so you need to use language that is literal and pre-
cise. The more detailed the message, the more "real" it
seems and the more easily the subconscious accepts it.

  NO: I will eat better.

  YES: I eat and enjoy five servings of fruits and vegetables
  a day.

  NO: I will rest more.

  YES: I lie down on the family room couch for thirty
  minutes every afternoon.

- **If possible, set measurable goals.** State a specific goals in a
quantifiable way. Specific targets are easier to achieve.

  NO: I will get more sleep.

  YES: I sleep eight hours a night.

- **Use motivating language.** The more enjoyable a suggestion sounds, the more likely it will be followed.

  NO: I will exercise every day.

  YES: I enjoy a thirty-minute walk every afternoon.

  NO: I will drink milk every day.

  YES: I enjoy drinking a glass of milk with every meal.

- **Make a choice.** Suggestions that include the words "I choose" can be very powerful.

  YES: I choose to feel relaxed and free from stress.

  YES: I choose to breathe only clean, smoke-free air for my baby.

- **Repeat your suggestion; repeat your suggestion.** Repetition helps drive the point home to the subconscious. Change the wording if you wish, but keep the content the same. Approach offering a hypnotic suggestion like an advertiser approaches buying commercial time: the more, the better. The more often your subconscious hears a message, the more it believes it.

- **Use "triggers" to strengthen hypnotic suggestions.** Triggers can be images, movement, or physical sensations that can be programmed into your subconscious to reinforce a hypnotic suggestion.

  EXAMPLE: Every time you see an infant, you relax and

feel confident that everything will go well with your pregnancy. You will soon meet your beloved baby face to face.

EXAMPLE: When you walk through the doors and enter the hospital, you will feel relaxed and comfortable. With every step you take, you will become more relaxed and confident that you and your baby will be healthy and safe.

EXAMPLE: Every time you sense your uterus contract, you feel more and more relaxed. You reach a deeper state of concentration and relaxation. Your body is preparing for delivery; it won't be long now.

Suggestions for Pain Control

You can use special suggestions to control pain during childbirth. Experiment with all of the techniques and choose the approach that works best for you. (For sample scripts of these techniques, see Chapter 5.)

- Glove anesthesia: This is the most common and most successful approach to pain control during childbirth. You alter the feelings in your hand by making it feel numb or tingling (this is fairly easy for most people to do). Then you are able to transfer the feeling of your hand to any part of your body you touch. During labor you will be able to relieve any discomfort in your abdomen by merely touching your hand to your body.

- Dissociation: This approach allows you to divorce yourself from your pain by changing it into something else. You might imagine your pain as a blue spot, then mentally shrink the size of the spot, and your pain vanishes at the same time. Or you can see it as a ship and have it sail off into the horizon. Or you can move the pain to another part of your body, gradually pushing it to the ends of your fingers and out of your body.

- Visualization: This technique builds on the fact that you cannot feel pain and pleasure at the same time. Minimize the pain by seeing yourself in a place that makes you feel calm, safe, and comfortable.

With practice, most people can use these suggestions to reach a deep enough state of hypnosis to experience anesthesia. (Anesthesia means the inability to feel anything; with the approach described here, you will lose all sensation in the affected part of your body.) The mind is a powerful tool, and you can use it to overcome pain. Visualization is effective because the same regions of the brain are stimulated whether a person is performing an activity or merely imagining it. To the brain, what is imagined can become real.

Is Your Hypnosis Really Working?

After practicing regularly for several weeks, it is a good idea to perform an experiment to prove to yourself that hypnosis for pain control will work for you. Have your partner bring you into a deepened state of hypnosis, then practice the pain control exercises while holding an ice cube in your hand for sixty seconds.

(Have your partner limit the time you hold the ice cube to simulate a "contraction.")

Once you have mastered this exercise, repeat the exercise but hold the ice cube against the inside of your wrist or behind your ear. This is a more intense type of sensation that takes more concentration to control. Finally, repeat the exercise again, this time holding two ice cubes, one in each hand (or one behind each ear) for sixty seconds. This is more difficult because the sensation involves two different locations on your body.

You can give yourself the ice cube test in an unhypnotized state, to appreciate just how effective hypnosis can be!

It's Time to Close

The final phase of hypnosis involves verbal instructions to exit the hypnotic trance. It is simple to broaden your attention and return to the normal state of awareness. Remember that you were the one who brought yourself to the state of relaxation, and you can snap out of it at will, even when you are in the deepest hypnotic state.

As you close the session, you choose what you want to remember about your time under hypnosis. When it comes to childbirth, you will not have experienced pain, so there are no painful memories to recall, but you can remember anything else about your labor and delivery.

The closing words are simple and short. The typical closing involves the suggestion to feel relaxed and refreshed when you come out of the trance. In most cases, the closing also includes a suggestion that it will be easier to enter hypnosis the next time and that the next hypnosis session will be very productive. After these final suggestions are made, you may be told to count out loud from one to three and open your eyes. (Sample language that can be used for a closing is included in Chapter 5.)

During labor, some women want to know what it feels like to experience a few contractions in the unhypnotized state. They cannot accept that hypnosis is as powerful a tool as it is, or they want to have the experience so that they know what other women are talking about. In any case, if you want to feel a contraction and perceive it in all its glory, you can prepare in advance a suggestion that brings you out of hypnosis very rapidly—and allows you to become rehypnotized just as quickly. For example, you might have the suggestion that you will come out of hypnosis if your partner touches your right shoulder, and you will reenter hypnosis if he touches your left shoulder. Or you can come up with a word or gesture that has the same effect.

The Importance of Practice

To be successful with hypnosis during childbirth, you have to practice at home. You can reinforce your suggestions by working with a partner or by using a tape-recorded message for self-hypnosis. In each session, you should include an induction, deepening, suggestions, and closure. (Each session should include some work with pain control, specifically the section on glove anesthesia.) You can use the scripts in the chapter that follows as they are written or modify them to help prepare for a joyful and painless childbirth.

5

■ ■ ■ ON YOUR OWN
Hypnosis Scripts You Can Practice
Without Professional Assistance

If you want to face labor and delivery without pain or anxiety, you need to practice the hypnosis skills outlined in this book. When working with a professional hypnotherapist, most sessions last about sixty to ninety minutes. However, when practicing self-hypnosis at home, expect to spend about twenty to thirty minutes every day. Remember, the more you practice, the more confident you will be when your baby's birthday arrives. There is no harm in practicing twice a day, if you want to work it into your routine.

It's best to make hypnosis a part of your daily routine. Try to set aside a period of uninterrupted time every day to work on your skills with a partner or with a tape recording. It is easier to hypnotize yourself if you have been hypnotized by someone else, but it is possible to do it all on your own.

This chapter includes scripts that your partner can read to you or that you can read into a tape recorder to prepare a tape for self-hypnosis. You can read them as written, edit them, or prepare your own.

When reading a script, use a relaxed, monotone voice. Don't rush the words. Try to enunciate clearly; you don't want your subconscious to misunderstand or to struggle to decipher mumbled words.

Some people find it helpful to have background music, the sound of ocean waves, or the steady beat of a metronome on the tape. The end of the music can help to indicate when the hypnosis session has ended. This is a matter of personal preference.

If you are preparing an audiotape to hypnotize yourself, you can choose whether to use the first person ("I") or the third person ("you") when making the suggestions. Both methods work well; again, it is a matter of personal preference.

If you are making tapes for self-hypnosis, include the entire script on a single tape so that you can play the tape without interruption. You can record different versions if you want to modify the session to address particular complaints during pregnancy, such as insomnia or leg cramps. Most tapes will run about sixty minutes or so.

You will use your tape to practice hypnosis in preparation for labor. If you are working with a partner or hypnotherapist, it is helpful to practice using both live and recorded sessions. The recordings can help you practice on your own, and the one-on-one sessions can help you build confidence in your relationship with your hypnosis partner, who will guide you during your actual labor.

Preparing Your Hypnosis Script

Before starting a hypnosis session, read through this entire chapter and choose which sample scripts seem most natural to you. Feel free to modify them or to write your own, using imagery that is meaningful to you. The more detailed you can be, the more effective the script will be.

For the hypnosis session, be sure you include an induction, a deepener, the suggestions, and a closing. For the first few weeks, experiment with different images and approaches. Your goal is to find the language that proves most effective at promoting relaxation and concentration. If any approach feels awkward or distracting, abandon it and try something else.

Induction Scripts

Here are several sample induction scripts. No matter which script you choose, you will begin to feel pleasantly relaxed as you follow the instructions of the hypnotist's voice.

Whenever possible, use detailed language that invokes as many of the senses as possible. When you imagine the beach, see the ocean waves, smell the suntan lotion, feel the warm sand between your toes, hear the cry of the seagulls, and taste the salty ocean mist. The more specific the image, the more effective it is for hypnosis.

Countdown

Sit back comfortably. Good. Now put your feet squarely on the floor and rest your hands on your lap.

Okay. Now take a slow, deep breath. Fill your lungs with fresh air. Hold it for a moment. Now exhale. Let the air go slowly, through your mouth. As you exhale, let all the tension you feel leave your body. Do it again. In . . . and out. Good. In . . . and out.

Now you're going to count backward from 30. You will count slowly and deliberately. As you do so, you will feel more and more relaxed. Okay. Let's get started.

30 . . .

29 . . . you feel very relaxed . . .

28 . . . 27 . . . your eyes are getting heavy . . .

26 . . . so heavy . . .

25 . . . so heavy you want to close them . . .

24 . . . 23 . . . it's hard to keep your eyes open, they feel so heavy . . .

22 . . . 21 . . . it's okay to close your eyes if you want . . .

20 . . . closing your eyes feels so relaxing . . .

19 . . . so peaceful. Your eyes are so heavy you must close them. It feels so good to close your eyes.

Another Option

You can count backward from 100 by 3s: 97, 94, 91, 88, 85. . . . This can be helpful if you are nervous about being hypnotized, because when your mind is focused on the computation it lets go of the anxiety.

Eye Fixation: Stare at an Imaginary Spot

Sit back comfortably. Take a slow, deep breath. Let it go. Breathe in again. This time let the tension leave your body as you exhale. Deep breath. In with fresh air. Now out with tension. You are relaxed.

Okay. Now that you are relaxed, I would like you to look at an imaginary spot on the ceiling above your forehead. Choose any spot and stare at it. Don't move your head, just your eyes. Let your eyes roll way back. Back, the farther the better, until they are on the spot on the ceiling.

Stare at the spot. Stare. . . . You notice that your eyelids are getting heavier . . .

and heavier . . .

and heavier.

Keep your eyes on the spot. Don't let them drift. You find it difficult to keep your eyes open. . . . When you allow them to close you will feel so relaxed. You want to close your eyes.

Another Option

You can stare at a candle flame.

Watch the Moving Object

Sit back comfortably. Inhale. Take a slow, deep breath. Fill your lungs with air. Good. Now let it go. Breathe in again, and this time let the tension leave your body as you exhale. Take a deep breath. Breathe in relaxation, breathe out tension. In with relaxation, out with tension.

Now it is time to really relax. Let your eyes follow the pocket watch. Look at it as it swings back and forth, back and forth. Notice the shiny gold as it goes back and forth.

Breathe in . . . back and forth. . . .

Breathe out . . . back and forth. . . .

Keep your eyes on the pocket watch as it goes back and

forth. You are so relaxed, so deeply relaxed. Each time the watch swings, you can feel yourself relaxing deeper and deeper.

Your eyes are beginning to feel heavy. Very heavy. . . .

Your eyelids are feeling so heavy that it is difficult to keep them open. . . .

You feel your eyelids closing. . . .

It's okay to allow your eyelids to close . . . because you are so relaxed. So peaceful.

Another Option

You can stare at a spiral or an optical illusion.

Progressive Relaxation

Sit back comfortably. As we get started, I want you to draw in a deep breath. Now let it go. Again. Fill your lungs with relaxing oxygen. And breathe out tension. Feel the tension leave your body as you exhale. Deep breath. In with fresh air. Now out with tension.

Now you are going to relax your entire body. As we work through this exercise, you will feel all of the tension drain from your body. You will start with your feet and work up to your scalp, growing more relaxed at each step.

I want you to focus on your toes. Tense your toes. Feel the muscles in your toes contract. Flex them tighter. Hold a moment . . . now relax them gradually. Feel the relaxation wash over your muscles as you release them. Allow those muscles to feel limp and wooden. They are completely relaxed.

Now move on to your calves. Focus on these muscles and then tense them. Feel the muscles in your calves contract. Tight, tighter. Feel the muscle pull against the bone. Hold it . . . hold. Now relax. A warm feeling of relaxation comes across the muscle. You feel relaxed, so relaxed it almost seems that these muscles are no longer a part of you.

Now your thighs. Extend your legs and flex the muscles in your thighs. Tense them. Flex them as tightly as you can. Tighter . . . tighter. Hold it . . . a moment . . . longer. Slowly release the muscle. Slowly allow those feelings of absolute relaxation to spread though your thighs, down your calves, and into your feet. You are relaxed, so relaxed.

Move up to your buttocks. Squeeze your buttocks together. Contract these muscles and hold them as tight as you can. Feel the squeeze. Tighter, tighter. Now relax them. Feel the warm rush of relaxation spread across your buttocks. Enjoy the calm, soothing feeling of relaxation.

Now your abdomen. You can feel the muscles that stretch across you abdomen. You can feel them stretch across your uterus where your baby lives. Tense those muscles. Feel your abdomen contract, just like you're pulling yourself up from a chair or doing a sit-up. Tighten those muscles. Tighter, tighter. Hold . . . that's right, hold it. Now release. Feel the muscles across your abdomen relax. It feels so good to let the tension go. It feels so good to relax.

Now let's move up to your fingers and hands. Focus all of your attention on your fingers and hands. Okay, now tense your fingers and hands. Squeeze them into a tight fist. Feel all the muscles contract and grow tighter, tighter.

Hold the fist. Squeeze your hands tighter, even tighter. Good. Now relax all of the muscles in your fingers and hands. Allow your fingers to unfold like a flower opening. Feel the tension melt away as your fingers relax. Your hands feel limp, heavy, wooden. They are completely relaxed.

Now focus on your arms. Tense all the muscles in your arms. Feel them flex and tighten. Flex them more . . . and more . . . and more. Now relax them. Slowly release the muscles and feel the wave of relaxation spread down your arms. Let your arms feel limp, heavy, free of any tension or tightness. Completely relaxed. Completely free from all stress.

Let's move on to your shoulders. Think about the muscles in your shoulders. Tense those muscles. Squeeze them as tight as you can. Tighter, tighter. Now hold . . . hold a little bit longer. Okay, now release. Again, feel the soothing sensation of relaxation as it spreads across your shoulders, down your back and arms. Allow the muscles in your shoulders to feel soft. So relaxed . . . they are completely relaxed.

Now your neck. Tense your neck muscles. Feel the strain as the muscles firmly but gently flex. Hold . . . hold . . . hold . . . now release. Feel the relaxation. So calm, so soothing.

Now your face. Scrunch up all the muscles in your face. Feel your face squeeze up tight, pucker your lips, and squeeze . . . squeeze. Hold it . . . hold it . . . hold. Now slowly relax. Feel your face grow softer and more relaxed. More relaxed than before. More relaxed than ever before.

Your entire body is relaxed now.

Your face ... all trace of tension is gone.

Your neck ... so relaxed, so calm.

Your shoulders ...

Your arms ...

Your hands and fingers ... You are limp, so relaxed you are unable to move. There is no need to move.

Your abdomen ...

Your buttocks ...

Your thighs ...

Your calves ... relaxed ...

Your toes ...

Everything is completely relaxed. Your body feels heavy, tranquil. You feel like a rag doll, soothed and relaxed.

The Skeptic's Induction

If you find it difficult to use the traditional inductions because you feel uncomfortable with the suggestions, try this approach. It uses physical sensations rather than mental imagery to focus the mind, making it a more effective approach for people who resist entering a trance.

Sit comfortably with your feet flat on the floor and the palms of your hands on your thighs. Take a deep breath in. Now exhale. Again, inhale. Exhale. Good. Now look at your hands. Stare at them. Really stare at them.

Press your palms down on your thighs. Harder. Push as if you are pressing your feet to the floor. Harder ... harder.

As you press, your fingers become more sensitive. Perhaps you can feel the warmth of your body under your clothes. Keep pressing. Harder.

As you press, notice that one of your fingers feels lighter than the rest. It may the pointer finger on your right hand. It may be the little finger of your left hand. You choose the finger. Feel the lightness. Keep pressing, pressing. It doesn't matter which finger feels lighter. If you really want to go into a deep state of relaxation, you will choose a finger, whichever one you want, and it will feel lighter. Concentrate. Think about the sensations in the finger.

Keep pressing, keep pressing. This finger, the lighter one, is beginning to twitch. Feel the muscles tremble, feel it twitch.

You want to lift this finger. Concentrate. You want to raise it above the others. Take your time. It is lighter than the rest. Keep pressing. It is up to you to decide when the finger will become lighter. It may happen in ten seconds . . .

or twenty seconds . . .

or thirty seconds . . . lighter . . . the finger is lighter . . .

You want to lift the finger. It's up to you to decide when to lift it . . .

Good. It feels so wonderful to let the finger get lighter and lighter. It is so relaxing. Concentrate on the finger. If you want to relax further, you can close your eyes and let the other fingers on your hand relax. Relax. Let all the fingers on the hand relax and lift off your thigh. They are so light they lift off your leg. As you release your finger, you feel more relaxed. As your hand rises, you become more relaxed . . .

lifting, lifting . . .
lighter, lighter . . .
more and more relaxed. . . .

Deepening Scripts

You have reached the first stage of hypnosis, and now it is time to go deeper. When you reach deeper levels of hypnosis, you still have absolute control over your behavior, of course, but you are so relaxed and so comfortable that it feels more satisfying to follow the suggestion of your tape than to try to resist.

Eyes Shut

Now, if you want to, you can reach a deeper state of relaxation. . . .

Just imagine that your eyes are heavy, very heavy. . . . You find it impossible to open your eyes, no matter how hard you try. . . . They are so heavy . . . you are so relaxed . . . your eyes are shut tight . . . so heavy . . . you cannot open them.

You can stop trying to open them. Just let yourself go completely relaxed. Let yourself relax. At the count of three, you will notice that your eyes are locked tight . . . and you are completely relaxed. . . .

One . . . your eyes are heavy and heavier. . . .

Two . . . your lids are heavy . . . you are so tired. It will feel so good to close your eyes. . . . Your eyes are closing . . . you are feeling more relaxed. . . .

Three . . . shut your eyes, tight, tighter. Let your eyes roll up into the back of your head, just like you are looking up at your hair. . . .

Keep your eyes shut and breathe in . . . slowly, naturally. Deep breath. You are feeling more relaxed with every breath. If you want, you can go deeper into relaxation with every breath . . .

Just listen to my voice . . .

Just relax.

Elevator

You are relaxed. Every bit of tension has left your body. It has been replaced with feelings of peace and warmth. . . .

Imagine that you have stepped into an elevator. As I count backward from ten, you will feel yourself becoming more and more relaxed. You feel the elevator begin to move.

Ten . . . let the tension leave your body.

Nine . . . tension is draining from your body. You have never felt this relaxed before. . . .

Eight . . . so calm, so peaceful . . .

Seven . . . you are still more relaxed . . .

Six . . . and more relaxed . . .

Five . . . the elevator is going down and you feel so heavy . . .

Four . . . so free from stress . . .

Three . . . we are getting near the bottom. . . .

Two . . . at the bottom you will feel completely relaxed. . . .

One . . . the elevator stops. You feel more relaxed than ever before. Completely at ease.

Another Option

If you don't like elevators, you can imagine yourself walking down steps, perhaps steps in a garden or steps down from a patio to a sunset on the beach. You could also walk along a long path with trees on either side, and with every step you become more relaxed.

Stepping into a Pool of Water

You feel relaxed and calm. A nice, soothing feeling of absolute relaxation is taking over your body. Feel it down at your toes. You feel as if your body is being dipped slowing into a warm pool of soothing, cleansing water.

When part of your body reaches the water, it is completely relaxed. That's right, start with your toes. Feel them relax. Feel the tension wash out of your body and into the water. You are so relaxed. You feel nothing but soothing warmth.

Now your calves are in the water. Feel the wave of relaxation soak into your body, up to your calves and thighs. You feel more and more relaxed. So relaxed you can't move, you don't want to move. The feeling is moving up, up.

Your legs feel heavy, calm. No need to move. Everything is heavy and relaxed. . . .

Now you feel that warmth and calm enter your fingertips. It feels warm, soothing. Feel it spread from your fingertips up your arms. The soothing feeling is soaking into your body, your fingers, your wrists, your arms, all the way up to your shoulders. Feel it reach your shoulders. So heavy, almost a detached feeling. Calm, so calm and relaxed.

Your arms feel so relaxed that they are almost numb. So heavy. Feel the calm spread to your abdomen and back. You feel completely relaxed, completely at ease.

Each breath you take makes you more relaxed. Every time you breathe in, you can feel yourself reach a deeper and deeper state of relaxation.

Relaxed . . . from head to toe . . .

Perfect peace.

Pick a Color, Any Color

You can give yourself the suggestion that you will experience a deeper state of relaxation every time you think of a certain color. This helps you slip into a deep state of relaxation very quickly. The color is yours to choose. Pick a shade that has a positive association for you.

Now I would like you to think of a cool blue. The color of a Caribbean sea. The color of a cloudless sky. Every time you think of that color, you will relax more.

Focus on the color. Feel yourself slip into a deeper and deeper state of relaxation.

Anytime you want to feel peaceful and relaxed, all you have to do is think of your color. That's right, see your color and feel that sense of peace and calm.

The Fading Numbers

You are relaxed, but now it is time to relax your mind as well as your body. So calm and deeply relaxed.

In a moment I am going to ask you to count backward from 100. With each number, you will feel deeper and deeper relaxed. Five times more relaxed than you were. So calm and so heavy.

When you say the number, either to yourself or out loud, I want you to visualize it in your mind. See the number while you feel more and more relaxed.

As you feel more relaxed, the number will fade away and the next number will appear.

You will find yourself so relaxed that all the numbers will disappear by the time you reach 96. You will be so relaxed that you will not be able to come up with any numbers. So calm, so peaceful. You will feel wonderful.

Okay, let's begin. 100 . . . you can feel yourself start to relax . . .

99 . . . deeper . . . and deeper . . .

98 . . . every bit of tension has drained from your body . . .

97 . . . every trace of stress is gone . . .

96 . . . you are so relaxed you cannot move, no need to move. You are in a state of perfect peace.

Suggestion Scripts

In this phase of hypnosis, you receive the suggestions that can deepen your state of relaxation and give you power over your perception of pain. Some people want suggestions that will help eliminate their pain; others want to escape discomfort; others want to lose themselves in the experience itself, perhaps by visualizing what is happening within their bodies as the baby is emerging. Experiment with different approaches to find one that is right for you.

You can use the following scripts as a starting point for you to write your own, incorporating imagery that is meaningful to you. You can be as creative as you wish with this part of the script.

Please keep in mind, however, that the suggestions must to be positive, stated in the present tense, specific, measurable, and motivating. Feel free to restate and repeat suggestions as often as necessary.

Glove Anesthesia

This approach will help you experience numbness that you can move around your body.

Imagine that you have in front of you a bucket containing a liquid that looks and smells like ice water. But this is special water. It is an anesthetic that soaks into the skin and makes whatever it touches feel numb.

Now take your right hand and slowly dip it into the bucket. Feel the anesthetic cover your fingertips. Feel the skin start to tingle as the fluid begins to work.

Dip your hand in up to your wrist. That's right. Now your entire hand is tingling. It is beginning to lose all sensation.

Lift your hand out of the bucket. It is completely numb. No feeling at all. It feels as if you dipped your hand in Novocain.

When I tell you to, place your hand on your abdomen. When your hand touches your abdomen, the anesthetic is transferred from your hand to your abdomen. Any sensation in your abdomen fades away . . . you cannot feel anything at all.

Return your hand to the bucket and soak up more of the numbing fluid. Move it to your abdomen again to add more anesthetic. You can do this anytime you wish, moving the numbing feeling from the bucket to your hand . . . from your hand to your abdomen. . . . It's up to you to allow the numbness to spread.

When you're ready to regain feeling, simply shake your hand. Shake the fluid off your hand.

First, the tingling sensation returns. Feel the tingle. . . .

Then you gain full sensation in your hand. Your hand feels just like it did before you put it in the bucket.

Dissociation

With this approach you imagine your pain as something else and you transform it using your imagination.

You are completely relaxed. So calm and relaxed. Imagine that you are looking at a clear, blue summer sky. A gentle breeze is blowing and you are completely relaxed.

Look, a dark storm is forming in the middle of the sky. The white cloud is becoming gray, darker and darker gray. All of your discomfort is in that cloud. All of your tension, all of your anxiety. Any feelings that you want to dismiss, they are all in the cloud, in the dark cloud in the middle of the sky.

Now watch as the wind grows stronger. The wind is building in intensity. It is now blowing away the cloud, blowing away the discomfort, blowing away the tension.

The cloud is beginning to spread out. See the dark cloud get lighter in color. See the cloud begin to move away.

Let it go . . . let the cloud blow away. Let it dissolve. Let the wind blow away any feelings of discomfort.

Just let it go. . . .

Let it go and feel more relaxed. More at ease.

Another Option

You are completely relaxed. So calm and relaxed. Imagine that you are looking at a pool of clear, blue water. In the middle of the pool is a small fish. See the scales, shimmering in the water. Watch the fish swim by.

All of the discomfort you feel is inside that small fish. See it swimming in a circle. Look, from the depth of the pool something is coming up from the water. It is a bigger fish. It has its mouth wide open. It is swimming toward the small fish.

Closer . . . closer. . . .

The big fish swallows the small fish. It then turns and dives back down into the water. The big fish is sinking deeper and deeper. . . .

The big fish is fading from sight. As the big fish disappears, so does all trace of discomfort. Let the big fish fade away. . . .

Just let it go. . . .

You feel calm, at peace. You are perfectly relaxed.

Another Option

You are completely relaxed. So calm, so peaceful. Imagine that you are in a tunnel. Turn one way and you can see the entrance. Turn the other way and you can see the exit.

Look toward the exit. You can see a light. The light is warm and bright and comforting. Take a step toward the light. . . .

Slowly walk toward the light. . . .

As you approach the light, you can feel your pain become less and less intense. . . .

The light seems to wash over you, making you feel calm and peaceful. . . .

With every step you feel more relaxed and comfortable. . . .

You are nearing the exit, and the pain is almost gone. . . .

You are bathed in the light . . . feel the warmth . . . you are free of all discomfort. . . .

You are perfectly relaxed. Perfectly at ease. Perfectly comfortable.

Other Ideas

• Imagine that you are on a ship. You see a box floating on the water. The box is holding your pain. Any feelings you don't want to experience have been stuffed into the box. The box begins to float away. As the box fades away, your pain disappears.

• Name the color of your pain. See the bright color of your discomfort begin to fade and lose intensity. As the color fades, so does the sensation of pain.

• Imagine your pain as a red dot. Feel the dot as a large spot, then gradually shrink the dot. Your pain is diminished as the dot shrinks in size. Eventually cause the dot—and the discomfort—to disappear.

• Visualize your pain as a blue mist. See it as a fog of light hazy blue. Take a deep breath, and as you exhale, allow the pain to be exhaled into the atmosphere, where it dissipates and disappears.

- Diminish your pain by mentally stretching your body. If you have pain in your abdomen, imagine your abdomen expanding like an inflated balloon. It is twice as big as it really is. With all of this additional room, your nerves and muscles no longer feel so tight.

Visualization

This technique allows you to imagine yourself in a soothing, comforting setting. You cannot feel pleasure and pain simultaneously, so you close out the experience of pain by maintaining a vivid mental image of a comfortable setting. It is essential to use as many of your senses as possible to make the exercise seem real.

Sit back comfortably. Take a slow, deep breath. Let it go. Breathe in again. Fill your lungs with fresh air. This time when you exhale, let all the tension leave your body. Deep breath in, relax. Exhale all the way, out with the tension.

You are completely relaxed. You are free from all care. Imagine that you are on your own private island.

This is your own special place. You are perfectly safe and sound. Nothing can happen on your island unless you want it to.

See yourself relaxing there. The white, sandy beach. The bright blue sky with fleecy white clouds. A summer sky. A line of palm trees near the beach offers a patch of shade.

Hear the sound of the waves lapping the sandy shore gently, rhythmically. Hear the waves. The rush of the water on the beach. The waves wash up to the beach with a whisper, then recede. Listen to the seagulls cry in the distance.

Smell the seaweed drying up on the shore. And the fragrance of suntan lotion, that unmistakable smell of summer. Taste the salty breeze. Feel the warm sand between your toes, so soothing and soft.

You are in a special place. You are safe and sound. You are relaxed. It is so peaceful here. So calm, so tranquil, so safe.

Another Option

Sit back and relax. Take a slow, deep breath. Exhale. Breathe in again. Fill your lungs, then exhale and release all of your tension. In with relaxation, out with tension.

You are relaxed and comfortable. Imagine that you are standing in a beautiful bathroom next to a freshly drawn bath. Scented candles are burning at the edge of the tub. Breathe in . . . smell the scent. Look at the candlelight reflect on the water.

Now imagine stepping into the warm water. Feel it wash over your feet and ankles. Imagine lowering yourself into the warm water. Not too hot, not too cold.

Lean back and feel the water wash over your body. You have never felt more relaxed. This is a special place. A place of perfect comfort. You feel calm, tranquil, safe.

Another Option

Take a deep breath, then let it go. Breathe in . . . and out. You are feeling completely relaxed. Breathe in . . . and out.

Imagine that you are lying in a hammock on a sunny afternoon. You are in a special place, where there are no worries. You are safe and sound. Nothing can happen to you when you are in your hammock, unless you want it to.

You feel relaxed in the hammock as it swings, ever so slightly, back and forth . . . back and forth. A gentle breeze is blowing. Feel it wash over you. The temperature is perfect . . . neither too hot nor too cold. You are so relaxed. . . .

It is so peaceful . . . you are calm, tranquil, safe.

Other Ideas

- You could be hiking on a forested path, walking among the enormous redwoods and watching the sun streak through the branches.

- You could be crawling into bed with fresh sheets after having worked in the garden all day. Your muscles are relaxed and you have enjoyed your day in the sunshine.

- Picture yourself floating on your back in the warm ocean waters of a Caribbean island. Feel the sun beating down, warming your body, and you feel light and calm.

Making Vacation Plans

When using visualization, be sure to choose a scene that you find peaceful and relaxing. Although many people find sitting on the beach relaxing, others fear the water and find the sand hot and uncomfortable. Some people enjoy an image of hiking through the woods on a cool fall afternoon, but others fear blistered feet, woodland ticks, and snakes crossing the dusty path. Be sure to think about which type of imagery is most relaxing to you and write your script around an idealized version of that experience.

Suggestion Script for Childbirth

During labor, it can be helpful to visualize images that reinforce the physical realities of what is happening to your body.

You are completely relaxed and comfortable. You feel joy and happiness because your baby will be born soon, very soon.

You can feel your uterus contract. It feels tight, but not too tight. You can feel the muscles gently squeeze to pull your cervix open. Let the muscles work. . . . When you feel a contraction, relax and feel your cervix relax and open . . . open so that your baby can come through. . . .

Every contraction brings the baby closer to you . . . every contraction brings your baby closer. . . .

When you feel the tightening, allow it to wash over you. You are floating on the wave of the contraction. . . . It carries you up, up . . . but it then fades away. . . .

Every contraction is a gift. . . . Every time your uterus tightens you are closer to delivery . . . closer to meeting your baby.

Imagine yourself with your baby. See yourself hold your baby for the first time. Feel your baby's weight against your arms. The soft skin. The gentle cry. Skin so smooth. You look down at your baby . . . those big clear eyes . . . and your baby looks back at you. . . .

You are calm and safe. Your baby will be here soon. . . .

Another Option

You are relaxed and comfortable. Your baby is on the way . . . your baby will be here soon, very soon.

You can feel your uterus contract. You can feel your muscles working to bring your baby into the world. Let these muscles do the work. . . .

Relax . . . let your cervix open . . . let your baby come to you. . . .

Imagine that your cervix is a flower. It is a bud that is slowly opening. . . .

With every contraction, you can see the flower open a little bit more. . . .

Your petals are opening, getting ready for your baby to slip through that opened flower. . . .

See the flower opening . . . wider, wider. . . .

When the flower is open, it will be time. It will be time

for your baby to be born. You are calm and safe. Your flower is opening.... Your baby will be here soon....

Time Distortion

You can give yourself the suggestion that time is passing more quickly than it actually is. In this way, your perception of the duration of labor is distorted by your mind.

You are completely relaxed. You feel joy because your baby will be here soon. Every ten minutes that pass will feel like one minute. Time has new meaning because you feel so much happiness. You are relaxed and joyful. You are eager to see your baby.

Enjoy Your Pregnancy

You can use hypnosis to reinforce certain positive attitudes about your pregnancy. You can also make suggestions about what it will be like and how much you will enjoy being a mother after your baby is born. Of course, these suggestions should follow induction and deepening.

You can feel your baby moving inside your uterus. You are the blessed carrier of a new life, the baby inside your body.

You want to take good care of yourself because you know that this is the way you can take care of your baby. You want to nourish your body by eating five servings of fruits and vegetables. You want to drink a glass of milk with every meal. You are responsible for eating foods that will nourish your baby as well as yourself.

You sleep well at night. You feel rested and refreshed when you wake up in the morning, ready for the day.

You exercise gently every day by walking for thirty minutes. You listen to the cues from your body, working hard enough to feel healthy without fatigue.

When it is time for your baby to be born, you will know just what to do. Your body will know just how to move. Trust your body. Trust your instincts. You will know how to move to feel comfortable. You will know when to push and when not to push. Everything will come easily to you.

You will feel safe and secure from the time you walk into the hospital to the time you leave. You are in good hands with the doctors and nurses. You can trust them to help you and your baby.

Imagine that you are in the delivery room at the hospital. Feel the love you have for your baby. Imagine that the feelings of love wash over your baby. The love will guide your baby, as the baby comes out of you, smoothly, gently.

Those feelings of love remind you that everything is okay. You are doing everything just right. You are safe. You are comfortable. You can trust your body.

Any time you want to during labor you can escape to a peaceful place. That's up to you. You can shut out anything you want by going to the place you have chosen. A place where you know you are calm and safe. You enjoy the feeling of the life inside you. You welcome the chance to bring your baby into the world. To hold your baby in your arms for the first time. You are privileged to be a mother. You will be a loving and nurturing mother. By loving your child you will love yourself. Take a deep breath. Imagine holding your baby in your arms. Feel the love you have for your child.

You can add other images to reinforce your role as a mother, or to assist with issues of concern after the baby is born. Here are a few suggestions.

• I am recovering rapidly from childbirth.

• I am a good mother. I enjoy nurturing my baby.

• Being a mother is the greatest joy I have ever known.

• I ask for help whenever I need it.

• I fall asleep easily when I choose to when the baby is napping.

• Feeding my baby is easy for me. I am relaxed at feeding time.

• I feel refreshed in the morning, even when I have been awake in the night.

- I cherish the moments I spend with my baby at night. Late-night feedings give me the opportunity to bond with my baby while the rest of the world sleeps.

- If someone else feeds the baby at night, I am able to sleep soundly through any disruptions. I trust that other people can love and care for my baby in the way that I do.

Success with Future Hypnosis Sessions

At the end of the suggestion phase of hypnosis, it is helpful to add a suggestion that you will find it easier to enter hypnosis and you will relax more deeply in the next session.

At your next hypnosis session you will find it easier to relax. You will become hypnotized more swiftly, and you will relax more deeply. You find hypnosis relaxing and beneficial.

Closure Scripts

You need to give your subconscious a signal that it is time to come out of the trance. This part of the session is usually relatively short.

In just a moment I will say the first four letters of the alphabet: A, B, C, and D. As I do so, you will begin to slowly open your eyes. Your eyes will be wide open when I reach letter D. You will feel relaxed and refreshed. You will look forward to the next hypnosis session, when you will reach a deeper state of relaxation. You will feel as if you just awakened from a restful night of sleep.

Okay. Listen now. A . . . it's time to gradually open your eyes. Slowly now. You feel relaxed, at peace.

B . . . your eyes open a little more now. . . . The next time you enter hypnosis, you will find it easier to reach an even deeper state of relaxation. . . .

C . . . you are feeling a bit more alert. You will soon resume your normal state of awareness. You feel refreshed and alert and look forward to the joyful celebration of your baby's birth. . . . You will be able to relax and remain relaxed through every contraction.

D . . . open your eyes and feel wonderful.

Another Option

You can substitute counting for the alphabet. You can also reverse the deepening message you used. For example, if you walked down a staircase, turn around and walk up the stairs. If you took an elevator to the tenth floor, push the button for the ground level and feel the elevator descend.

Short and Sweet Suggestions

Some people find minihypnosis sessions helpful for producing relaxation. In this simple approach, created by German psychiatrist Dr. J. H. Schultz, you simply sit in a comfortable position with your hands resting at your sides, close your eyes, and deliberately and slowly say to yourself:

I . . . am . . . relaxed.

I . . . am . . . relaxed.

I . . . am . . . relaxed.

You close by taking a deep breath and getting on with the day. The entire minisession should take about one minute and can be practiced three or more times a day.

This approach won't give you the specialized skills required for pain-free delivery, but it will help you remain relaxed. You can use it for other simple, direct suggestions. It can be very helpful in overcoming bad habits or instilling positive habits.

Success

After reading these scripts, you may find that some approaches feel more natural to you. You may use them as written or create one of your own. There are no special words that must be used for every person. The goal is to create a state of profound, focused relaxation.

Practice is essential because it trains your subconscious to accept the hypnotic suggestions without hesitation. Each time you hypnotize yourself, you are able to reach the same state of relaxation faster and more effectively. When your labor begins, you want to be ready to relax and enter hypnosis swiftly and with confidence. With practice, the desired effects of relaxation and anesthesia will be almost instantaneous.

When the moment arrives and you go into labor, stay calm and follow the simple guidelines.

- Start with relaxation. If you begin to feel anxious, have your partner bring you into a light trance to promote feelings of relaxation. Remain focused on your labor and the fact that you will meet your baby soon. You can remain in this light trancelike state as long as you feel relaxed and comfortable.

- When the contractions become more intense, introduce imagery designed to control pain. During this phase, your partner should use some of the exercises designed to minimize discomfort, while also helping you remain calm and peaceful. The more relaxed you feel, the easier your labor will be.

- When you enter the pushing phase of labor, your partner can support you by providing you with visual imagery to promote delivery.

Don't become too dependent on specific scripts. A successful partner can adapt the words to meet your immediate physical needs. For example, your partner might draw on physical cues from the delivery room by focusing on the weather outside the room or a piece of music playing. Both you and your partner need to be creative and flexible.

You can make hypnosis work for you. All you need to do is decide that you want to be hypnotized, pay attention and follow the hypnotic suggestions, and use your imagination. Remember that hypnosis is an exercise not of the will but of the imagination. You won't feel fundamentally different— just very relaxed—when you are in a hypnotic trance. If you choose to allow hypnosis to work for you, you are already on your way to a pain-free childbirth.

6

■ ■ ■ BEFORE THE BIRTH
*Treating the Common Complaints of
Pregnancy*

Most women experience some aches, pains, and complaints during pregnancy well before they go into labor. Hypnosis can be used to manage these gripes.

This chapter will help you use hypnosis to work through a number of common complaints of pregnancy, including headaches, heartburn, insomnia, leg cramps, morning sickness, and excessive weight gain.

Headaches

Many women find that they are more susceptible to headaches during pregnancy. Even though a quick trip to the medicine cabinet can cure most headaches when you're not pregnant, it's best to avoid most medicines when pregnant. The best solution: prevention.

Headaches during pregnancy are usually caused by hormonal changes, fatigue, stress (both physical and emotional), and hunger. You can prevent some headaches by doing your best to relax (and you know hypnosis can help), rest (especially during the first and third trimesters), and eat regularly (low blood sugar caused by skipped meals can trigger headaches).

Some women who suffer from migraine headaches report more frequent migraines during pregnancy, and others find that these throbbing, blinding headaches occur less often. The exact reason for this change in frequency is related to the myriad hormonal changes that occur throughout pregnancy. Physiologically, the problem involves the constriction of blood vessels in the head, followed by their sudden opening or dilation. In addition to debilitating pain, a migraine headache can be accompanied by nausea, vomiting, diarrhea, and sensitivity to light. The intense pain can strike one side of the head or both, or transfer from one side to the other.

Experiencing chronic headaches or your first migrainelike headache during pregnancy can be a sign of pregnancy-induced hypertension, a serious condition that needs prompt medical attention from your doctor. If you experience a headache that lasts for more than two hours, or if you experience puffiness and water retention in your hands and feet and visual disturbances (spots in front of your eyes), contact your obstetrician or health-care provider as soon as possible. However, for everyday headaches that tend to come and go, consider using hypnosis to help manage the discomfort.

Induction and Deepening
You may use the following induction script or choose another from Chapter 5.

Sit back comfortably. Good. Now put your feet squarely on the floor and rest your hands on your lap.

Okay. Now take a slow, deep breath. Fill your lungs with fresh air. Hold it for a moment. Now exhale. Let the air go slowly, through your mouth. As you exhale, let all the tension you feel leave your body. Do it again. In . . . and out. Good. In . . . and out.

Now you're going to count backward from 30. You will count slowly and deliberately. As you do so, you will feel more and more relaxed. Okay. Let's get started.

30 . . .

29 . . . you feel very relaxed . . .

28 . . . 27 . . . your eyes are getting heavy . . .

26 . . . so heavy . . .

25 . . . so heavy you want to close them . . .

24 . . . 23 . . . it's hard to keep your eyes open, they feel so heavy . . .

22 . . . 21 . . . it's okay to close your eyes if you want . . .

20 . . . closing your eyes feels so relaxing . . .

19 . . . so peaceful. Your eyes are so heavy you must close them. It feels so good to close your eyes.

Good. Very good.

Now if you want to, you can reach a deeper state of relaxation. . . .

Just imagine that your eyes are heavy, very heavy. . . . You find it impossible to open your eyes, no matter how hard you try. . . . They are so heavy . . . you are so relaxed . . . your eyes are shut tight . . . so heavy . . . you cannot open them.

You can stop trying to open them. Just let yourself go completely relaxed. Let yourself relax. At the count of

*three, you will notice that your eyes are locked tight . . .
and you are completely relaxed. . . .*

One . . . your eyes are heavy and heavier. . . .

*Two . . . your lids are heavy . . . you are so tired. It will
feel so good to close your eyes . . . Your eyes are closing . . .
you are feeling more relaxed. . . .*

*Three . . . shut your eyes, tight, tighter. Let your eyes roll
up into the back of your head, just like you are looking up
at your hair. . . .*

*Keep your eyes shut and breathe in . . . slowly, natu-
rally. Deep breath. You are feeling more relaxed with every
breath. If you want, you can go deeper into relaxation with
every breath. . . .*

Just listen to my voice. . . .

Just relax.

Suggestion

If you experience frequent headaches during pregnancy, you
may want to include a suggestion about headache relief in
your regular hypnosis session.

*You feel completely relaxed now. So calm and peaceful.
This feeling of relaxation will stay with you throughout
the day. When you begin to feel stress, all you have to do
is think of this feeling, and all the stress will drain away,
right out of your body. You will feel as if someone pulled
a plug and all the stress and tension just drain right out
of you.*

You take time to rest each day. You go to sleep each

night at your regular bedtime and you sleep peacefully through the night. You feel rested and refreshed when you wake up in the morning, ready to face a new day. You are pleased and excited at being one day closer to meeting your baby. You will soon be able to welcome your baby to the world.

If you feel any discomfort in your head, you will consciously relax yourself. You will take in a deep breath, and then let it go. When you do this, you will feel the discomfort drain away. Because you are relaxed. So calm and peaceful. In with refreshing, relaxing air . . . out with tension and stress. In with relaxation, out with tension. So calm . . . so peaceful.

Closing

You can use the following script or one of the others described in Chapter 5.

In just a moment I will say the first four letters of the alphabet: A, B, C, and D. As I do so, you will begin to slowly open your eyes. Your eyes will be wide open when I reach letter D. You will feel relaxed and refreshed. You will look forward to the next hypnosis session when you will reach a deeper state of relaxation. You will feel as if you just awakened from a restful night of sleep.

Okay. Listen now. A . . . it's time to gradually open your eyes. Slowly now. You feel relaxed, at peace.

B . . . your eyes open a little more now. . . . The next time you enter hypnosis, you will find it easier to reach an even deeper state of relaxation. . . .

C . . . you are feeling a bit more alert. You will soon resume your normal state of awareness. You feel refreshed and alert and look forward to the joyful celebration of your baby's birth. . . . You will be able to relax and remain relaxed through every contraction.

D . . . open your eyes and feel wonderful.

Heartburn

About two out of every three pregnant women suffer from heartburn or indigestion, especially during the third trimester. Heartburn is characterized by a burning sensation in the upper abdomen, throat, or lower part of the chest. Although this common complaint can make you quite uncomfortable, it does not hurt your baby in any way.

Heartburn and indigestion can occur whether at any time, but pregnancy cause a woman's body to produce high levels of progesterone and estrogen, which tend to relax smooth-muscle tissue, including the muscles in the gastrointestinal tract. When these muscles work less effectively, food tends to move through the body more slowly, which gives your body more time to extract nutrients. The problem arises because the ring of muscle that separates the esophagus from the stomach relaxes, allowing digestive acids to back up from the stomach into the esophagus. The acids burn the lining of the esophagus, causing a painful sensation. In late pregnancy, the problem is made worse when the uterus crowds the stomach, leaving it little room for expansion.

You can minimize your risk of heartburn by limiting weight gain, avoiding tight clothing, eating frequent small meals rather than fewer large ones, eating slowly, and sleeping with your head slightly elevated with an extra pillow. (Avoid taking antacids containing sodium or sodium bicarbonate during pregnancy.)

It also is essential that you relieve anxiety and tension to manage heartburn in pregnancy. Most women can do this with relaxation exercises or hypnosis. The following hypnosis script can help you reduce anxiety and put out the fires of indigestion.

Induction and Deepening
You may use the following induction script or choose another from Chapter 5.

> *Sit back comfortably. Good. Now put your feet squarely on the floor and rest your hands on your lap.*
>
> *Okay. Now take a slow, deep breath. Fill your lungs with fresh air. Hold it for a moment. Now exhale. Let the air go slowly, through your mouth. As you exhale, let all the tension you feel leave your body. Do it again. In . . . and out. Good. In . . . and out.*
>
> *Now you're going to count backward from 30. You will count slowly and deliberately. As you do so, you will feel more and more relaxed. Okay. Let's get started.*
>
> *30 . . .*
> *29 . . . you feel very relaxed . . .*
> *28 . . . 27 . . . your eyes are getting heavy . . .*
> *26 . . . so heavy . . .*
> *25 . . . so heavy you want to close them . . .*

24 . . . 23 . . . it's hard to keep your eyes open, they feel so heavy . . .

22 . . . 21 . . . it's okay to close your eyes if you want . . .

20 . . . closing your eyes feels so relaxing . . .

19 . . . so peaceful. Your eyes are so heavy you must close them. It feels so good to close your eyes.

Good. Very good.

Now, if you want to, you can reach a deeper state of relaxation. . . .

Just imagine that your eyes are heavy, very heavy. . . . You find it impossible to open your eyes, no matter how hard you try. . . . They are so heavy . . . you are so relaxed . . . your eyes are shut tight . . . so heavy . . . you cannot open them.

You can stop trying to open them. Just let yourself go completely relaxed. Let yourself relax. At the count of three, you will notice that your eyes are locked tight . . . and you are completely relaxed. . . .

One . . . your eyes are heavy and heavier. . . .

Two . . . your lids are heavy . . . you are so tired. It will feel so good to close your eyes. . . . Your eyes are closing . . . you are feeling more relaxed. . . .

Three . . . shut your eyes, tight, tighter. Let your eyes roll up into the back of your head, just like you are looking up at your hair. . . .

Keep your eyes shut and breathe in . . . slowly, naturally. Deep breath. You are feeling more relaxed with every breath. If you want, you can go deeper into relaxation with every breath. . . .

Just listen to my voice. . . .
Just relax.

Suggestion

If you experience heartburn at a particular time of day, such as in the evening after dinner, you might want to try hypnosis for relaxation before heartburn strikes. If you are too late, the following suggestion might help.

You feel relaxed and at peace. When you feel the burning sensation of heartburn, you put out the flame by focusing on keeping the acids in your stomach. You will breathe in cool, fresh air . . . then breathe out any tension. Good. Breathe in air that will extinguish the fire . . . breathe out all stress and anxiety.

During the day, you eat a number of smaller meals rather than three large ones. You keep nutritious foods in your stomach without overeating. You enjoy mealtimes and take your time when eating. You savor every bite of food and stop eating when full.

Take a deep breath. Good. Now relax your esophagus. Feel the stomach acids retreat back into your stomach. Feel the burn disappear. Inhale. Now exhale. Feel all the heartburn pain wash away. You are calm. You are relaxed.

Closing

You can use the following script or one of the others described in Chapter 5.

In just a moment I will say the first four letters of the alphabet: A, B, C, and D. As I do so, you will begin to slowly open your eyes. Your eyes will be wide open when I reach letter D. You will feel relaxed and refreshed. You will look forward to the next hypnosis session, when you will reach a deeper state of relaxation. You will feel as if you just awakened from a restful night of sleep.

Okay. Listen now. A . . . it's time to gradually open your eyes. Slowly now. You feel relaxed, at peace.

B . . . your eyes open a little more now. . . . The next time you enter hypnosis, you will find it easier to reach an even deeper state of relaxation. . . .

C . . . you are feeling a bit more alert. You will soon resume your normal state of awareness. You feel refreshed and alert and look forward to the joyful celebration of your baby's birth. . . . You will be able to relax and remain relaxed through every contraction.

D . . . open your eyes and feel wonderful.

Insomnia

Many women experience insomnia to some degree during pregnancy. Some experts believe the tossing and turning at night is caused by hormonal changes; others think psychological factors and anxiety play the greatest role. Insomnia may respond to simple changes in behavior, such as getting enough exercise (but not too close to bedtime), eating at an unhurried pace, developing a bedtime routine, having a late-night snack to maintain stable blood-sugar levels at night, inhaling fresh air before bed, limiting fluids after 4 P.M. to reduce the number of trips to the bathroom, and relaxing. Of course, you should restrict caffeinated beverages to the morning hours, or eliminate them altogether.

Although these techniques can be helpful, insomnia also responds well to hypnosis. You are not asleep when you are in a hypnotic trance, but suggestions made while you are in a hypnotic trance can help you get to sleep.

Induction and Deepening

You may use the following induction script or choose another from Chapter 5.

Lie down and take a slow, deep breath. Fill your lungs with fresh air. Hold it for a moment. Now exhale. Let the air go slowly, through your mouth. As you exhale, let all the tension you feel leave your body. Do it again. In . . . and out. Good. In . . . and out.

Now you're going to count backward from 30. You will count slowly and deliberately. As you do so, you will feel more and more relaxed. Okay. Let's get started.

30 . . .

29 . . . you feel very relaxed . . .

28 . . . 27 . . . your eyes are getting heavy . . .

26 . . . so heavy . . .

25 . . . so heavy you want to close them . . .

24 . . . 23 . . . it's hard to keep your eyes open, they feel so heavy . . .

22 . . . 21 . . . it's okay to close your eyes if you want.

20 . . . closing your eyes feels so relaxing . . .

19 . . . so peaceful. Your eyes are so heavy you must close them. It feels so good to close your eyes.

Good. Very good.

Now if you want to, you can reach a deeper state of relaxation . . .

Just imagine that your eyes are heavy, very heavy. . . . You find it impossible to open your eyes, no matter how hard you try. . . . They are so heavy . . . you are so relaxed . . . your eyes are shut tight . . . so heavy . . . you cannot open them.

You can stop trying to open them. Just let yourself go completely relaxed. Let yourself relax. At the count of three, you will notice that your eyes are locked tight . . . and you are completely relaxed. . . .

One . . . your eyes are heavy and heavier . . .

Two . . . your lids are heavy . . . you are so tired. It will feel so good to close your eyes. . . . Your eyes are closing . . . you are feeling more relaxed. . . .

Three . . . shut your eyes, tight, tighter. Let your eyes roll up into the back of your head, just like you are looking up at your hair. . . .

Keep your eyes shut and breathe in . . . slowly, naturally. Deep breath. You are feeling more relaxed with every breath. If you want, you can go deeper into relaxation with every breath. . . .

Just listen to my voice. . . .

Just relax.

Suggestion

The relaxation exercises used in hypnosis can help you clear your mind and prepare for a night of restful sleep. This suggestion can be made during a regular hypnosis session, not before going to bed.

You feel completely relaxed and comfortable. When you climb into your bed at night, you still remember how this feels and relax the same way.

You have nothing to worry about. You are safe and sound. You will be holding your baby soon, and everything will be okay.

Breathe in . . . you are safe and sound.

Breathe out . . . you are safe and sound.

In . . . safe and sound . . .

Out . . . safe and sound . . .

When your regular bedtime comes, you will fall into a deep, relaxed sleep. When going to sleep, you will ignore all extraneous noises. You will enjoy a restful sleep and awaken feeling refreshed and energized.

You feel comfortable and tranquil. You allow sleep to overcome you. Just keep breathing in . . . safe and sound . . . and you will drift off to sleep.

You will stay asleep until morning, unless you must awaken at night. If you do wake up, it will be easy for you to get back to sleep. In fact, as soon as your head reaches the pillow and you close your eyes, you will fall asleep. Sound asleep. You are safe and sound . . . so sleepy . . . sleep.

Closing

You can use the following script or one of the others described in Chapter 5.

> *In just a moment I will say the first four letters of the alphabet: A, B, C, and D. As I do so, you will begin to slowly open your eyes. Your eyes will be wide open when I reach letter D. You will feel relaxed and refreshed. You will look forward to the next hypnosis session, when you will reach a deeper state of relaxation. You will feel as if you just awakened from a restful night of sleep.*
>
> *Okay. Listen now. A . . . it's time to gradually open your eyes. Slowly now. You feel relaxed, at peace.*
>
> *B . . . your eyes open a little more now. . . . The next time you enter hypnosis, you will find it easier to reach an even deeper state of relaxation. . . .*
>
> *C . . . you are feeling a bit more alert. You will soon resume your normal state of awareness. You feel refreshed and alert and look forward to the joyful celebration of your baby's birth. . . . You will be able to relax and remain relaxed through every contraction.*
>
> *D . . . open your eyes and feel wonderful.*

Another Option

If this approach does not work, you can trick yourself into falling asleep by telling yourself you cannot sleep. You can play this mind game with yourself while you are lying in bed preparing for sleep.

> *You are a night watchman on your rounds. It is dark outside and everything is quiet. You are not allowed to go*

to sleep while on your watch, but your eyes are getting heavy. You tell yourself that your eyes must remain open, but they are getting heavy, so heavy.

You want to blink your eyes, but each time you blink them your eyes get heavier and heavier. You try not to blink, but your eyelids feel like lead. So heavy. You blink and then you cannot stop from blinking. You simply must give in and close your eyes. It will be okay to close your eyes, if you want to. So heavy, so relaxed.

Leg Cramps

Leg cramps tend to strike late at night, when you least expect them. In many pregnant women, these muscle spasms are triggered by an excess of phosphorus and a shortage of calcium in the blood. Some experts believe that fatigue and the pressure of the expanding uterus can also cause cramping. If you experience cramps, elevate your legs for about thirty minutes a day, but also take time for about thirty minutes of gentle exercise, such as walking.

If you develop a cramp in your calf, flex your ankle and toes upward to stretch the muscle. Try standing on a cold surface as well. You may be able to use hypnosis to relax the muscles before they spasm, or to get them settled once a cramp begins. The following hypnosis script may help.

Induction and Deepening
You may use the following induction script or choose another from Chapter 5.

Sit back comfortably. Good. Now put your feet squarely on the floor and rest your hands on your lap.

Okay. Now take a slow, deep breath. Fill your lungs with fresh air. Hold it for a moment. Now exhale. Let the air go slowly, through your mouth. As you exhale, let all the tension you feel leave your body. Do it again. In . . . and out. Good. In . . . and out.

Now you're going to count backward from 30. You will count slowly and deliberately. As you do so, you will feel more and more relaxed. Okay. Let's get started.

30 . . .

29 . . . you feel very relaxed . . .

28 . . . 27 . . . your eyes are getting heavy . . .

26 . . . so heavy . . .

25 . . . so heavy you want to close them . . .

24 . . . 23 . . . it's hard to keep your eyes open, they feel so heavy . . .

22 . . . 21 . . . it's okay to close your eyes if you want . . .

20 . . . closing your eyes feels so relaxing . . .

19 . . . so peaceful. Your eyes are so heavy you must close them. It feels so good to close your eyes.

Good. Very good.

Now, if you want to, you can reach a deeper state of relaxation. . . .

Just imagine that your eyes are heavy, very heavy. . . . You find it impossible to open your eyes, no matter how hard you try. . . . They are so heavy . . . you are so relaxed . . . your eyes are shut tight . . . so heavy . . . you cannot open them.

You can stop trying to open them. Just let yourself go

completely relaxed. Let yourself relax. At the count of three, you will notice that your eyes are locked tight . . . and you are completely relaxed. . . .

One . . . your eyes are heavy and heavier. . . .

Two . . . your lids are heavy . . . you are so tired. It will feel so good to close your eyes . . . Your eyes are closing . . . you are feeling more relaxed. . . .

Three . . . shut your eyes, tight, tighter. Let your eyes roll up into the back of your head, just like you are looking up at your hair . . .

Keep your eyes shut and breathe in . . . slowly, naturally. Deep breath. You are feeling more relaxed with every breath. If you want, you can go deeper into relaxation with every breath . . .

Just listen to my voice . . .

Just relax.

Suggestion

If you develop chronic leg cramps, you can give yourself a suggestion to handle them by slipping right into hypnosis.

You are completely relaxed now. So calm and peaceful. You enjoy this feeling of comfort and relaxation. You will experience this same feeling of deep relaxation whenever you feel a leg cramp coming on. When you feel the muscle growing tighter, you will allow it to relax. Your whole body will feel calm. Your leg will feel relaxed.

When you feel the muscle in your leg tightening, you will slap the muscle a couple of times. When you do this, you will remind the muscle that it is time to relax. You will feel as calm and peaceful as you do right now. You will then focus your attention on the contracting muscle. When you do, you will feel it begin to relax.

You will be able to use your mind to imagine that you are dipping your leg in a pool of soothing warm water. As the leg enters the water, all the tension in it disappears. You can feel the muscle loosen and relax. Relax. So calm. When the muscle feels tight, you will use your imagination to put it in warm water, and it will relax. So comfortable. So calm. So relaxed.

Closing

You can use the following script or one of the others described in Chapter 5.

In just a moment I will say the first four letters of the alphabet: A, B, C, and D. As I do so, you will begin to slowly open your eyes. Your eyes will be wide open when I reach letter D. You will feel relaxed and refreshed. You will look forward to the next hypnosis session, when you will reach a deeper state of relaxation. You will feel as if you just awakened from a restful night of sleep.

Okay. Listen now. A . . . it's time to gradually open your eyes. Slowly now. You feel relaxed, at peace.

B . . . your eyes open a little more now. . . . The next time you enter hypnosis, you will find it easier to reach an even deeper state of relaxation. . . .

C . . . you are feeling a bit more alert. You will soon resume your normal state of awareness. You feel refreshed and alert and look forward to the joyful celebration of your baby's birth. . . . You will be able to relax and remain relaxed through every contraction.

D . . . open your eyes and feel wonderful.

Morning Sickness

Morning sickness is a misnomer; it can strike any time of the day or night. About half of all pregnant women experience morning sickness to some degree, typically during the first trimester. In rare cases, women develop hyperemesis—vomiting severe enough to require medical intervention.

In most cases the symptoms disappear without treatment by the fourth or fifth month of pregnancy, when the body has adjusted to the hormone imbalance caused by the pregnancy. The problem tends to be more severe and long-lasting in women carrying multiples.

No one knows the exact cause of morning sickness, but many experts suspect that both physical and psychological factors are involved. Studies have found that women with morning sickness tend to be easily hypnotized. Morning sickness is most common in first pregnancies, when the body is less prepared for the dramatic hormonal changes of pregnancy and the mind is less prepared for the monumental changes a woman faces when becoming a mother.

Common remedies include eating a diet high in protein and complex carbohydrates, drinking lots of water and other fluids, avoiding foods that make you feel queasy, eating often rather than waiting for hunger to strike, nibbling food before getting out of bed to raise blood-sugar levels before rising, getting extra sleep and relaxation, and minimizing stress.

If you think about feeling nauseated, the condition can be made worse. In the same way, you can use your mind to make the condition better, and hypnosis can help. Following is a hypnosis script designed to help manage morning sickness.

Induction and Deepening
You may use the following induction script or choose another from Chapter 5.

Sit back comfortably. Good. Now put your feet squarely on the floor and rest your hands on your lap.

Okay. Now take a slow, deep breath. Fill your lungs with fresh air. Hold it for a moment. Now exhale. Let the air go slowly, through your mouth. As you exhale, let all the tension you feel leave your body. Do it again. In . . . and out. Good. In . . . and out.

Now you're going to count backward from 30. You will count slowly and deliberately. As you do so, you will feel more and more relaxed. Okay. Let's get started.

30 . . .

29 . . . you feel very relaxed . . .

28 . . . 27 . . . your eyes are getting heavy . . .

26 . . . so heavy . . .

25 . . . so heavy you want to close them . . .

24 . . . 23 . . . it's hard to keep your eyes open, they feel so heavy . . .

22 . . . 21 . . . it's okay to close your eyes if you want.

20 . . . closing your eyes feels so relaxing . . .

19 . . . so peaceful. Your eyes are so heavy you must close them. It feels so good to close your eyes.

Good. Very good.

Now if you want to, you can reach a deeper state of relaxation. . . .

Just imagine that your eyes are heavy, very heavy. . . . You find it impossible to open your eyes, no matter how hard you try. . . . They are so heavy . . . you are so relaxed . . . your eyes are shut tight . . . so heavy . . . you cannot open them.

You can stop trying to open them. Just let yourself go completely relaxed. Let yourself relax. At the count of three, you will notice that your eyes are locked tight . . . and you are completely relaxed. . . .

One . . . your eyes are heavy and heavier. . . .

Two . . . your lids are heavy . . . you are so tired. It will feel so good to close your eyes. . . . Your eyes are closing . . . you are feeling more relaxed. . . .

Three . . . shut your eyes, tight, tighter. Let your eyes roll up into the back of your head, just like you are looking up at your hair. . . .

Keep your eyes shut and breathe in . . . slowly, naturally. Deep breath. You are feeling more relaxed with every breath. If you want you can go deeper into relaxation with every breath. . . .

Just listen to my voice. . . .

Just relax.

Suggestion

You can use this suggestion as part of your daily hypnosis practice session if you have problems with morning sickness.

You feel relaxed and comfortable. Your stomach feels calm. You are satisfied.

Now imagine seeing a plate of your favorite healthful foods. Imagine taking your first bite and enjoying it. It tastes better than anything you have ever tasted before. You can smell the food and taste it without feeling the slightest bit queasy. You want to eat nutritious foods. You want to choose nourishing foods for you and for your baby. You enjoy eating healthful foods. Your stomach feels satisfied and relaxed after eating.

Closing

You can use the following script or one of the others described in Chapter 5.

In just a moment I will say the first four letters of the alphabet: A, B, C, and D. As I do so, you will begin to slowly open your eyes. Your eyes will be wide open when I reach letter D. You will feel relaxed and refreshed. You will look forward to the next hypnosis session, when you will reach a deeper state of relaxation. You will feel as if you just awakened from a restful night of sleep.

Okay. Listen now. A . . . it's time to gradually open your eyes. Slowly now. You feel relaxed, at peace.

B . . . your eyes open a little more now. . . . The next time you enter hypnosis, you will find it easier to reach an even deeper state of relaxation. . . .

C . . . you are feeling a bit more alert. You will soon resume your normal state of awareness. You feel refreshed

and alert and look forward to the joyful celebration of your
baby's birth. . . . You will be able to relax and remain re-
laxed through every contraction.

  D . . . open your eyes and feel wonderful.

Weight Gain (Excessive)

Weight gain is an inevitable part of pregnancy, but excessive weight gain is not. Being pregnant does not give you carte blanche to eat as much as you want of whatever foods you want to eat. In fact, pregnancy is a time to be very careful with the foods you choose. After all, the foods you eat are nourishing not only you but your baby as well.

Most women should gain between twenty-five and thirty-five pounds during pregnancy. Gaining less than twenty pounds can result in a baby that is born premature, small, and less developed than he or she would be if properly nourished. Gaining excess weight can make the baby grow to the point that vaginal delivery becomes difficult, and the excess weight can be difficult to lose after delivery.

Weight gain alone, however, does not solely determine the size of your baby. Some women gain forty to fifty pounds and deliver six-pound babies, whereas other women barely gain twenty pounds and give birth to solid, eight-pound infants. The more important factor is the quality of the foods you eat. Your goal during pregnancy—and even when you're not pregnant—is to eat a balanced diet with an emphasis on healthful foods, especially fresh fruits and vegetables.

When assessing your weight gain, consider that six to eight pounds of the weight you're carrying is the baby itself. Another fourteen to twenty-four pounds is the placenta, amniotic fluid, blood, increase in breast and uterine tissue, and nominal increase in maternal fat (the reserves are designed to be used up during breast-feeding).

In most cases, women gain about three or four pounds during the first trimester, twelve to fourteen pounds during the second trimester, and eight to ten pounds during the third trimester. Some women stop gaining weight during the last few weeks of pregnancy. If you are gaining weight faster than recommended, discuss the matter with your obstetrician or health-care provider. You can also use hypnosis to reinforce the importance of eating regular, nutritious meals.

Induction and Deepening

You may use the following induction script or choose another from Chapter 5.

Sit back comfortably. Good. Now put your feet squarely on the floor and rest your hands on your lap.

Okay. Now take a slow, deep breath. Fill your lungs with fresh air. Hold it for a moment. Now exhale. Let the air go slowly, through your mouth. As you exhale, let all the tension you feel leave your body. Do it again. In . . . and out. Good. In . . . and out.

Now you're going to count backward from 30. You will count slowly and deliberately. As you do so, you will feel more and more relaxed. Okay. Let's get started.

30 . . .

29 . . . you feel very relaxed . . .

28 . . . 27 . . . your eyes are getting heavy . . .

26 . . . so heavy . . .

25 . . . so heavy you want to close them . . .

24 . . . 23 . . . it's hard to keep your eyes open, they feel so heavy . . .

22 . . . 21 . . . it's okay to close your eyes if you want . . .

20 . . . closing your eyes feels so relaxing . . .

19 . . . so peaceful. Your eyes are so heavy you must close them. It feels so good to close your eyes.

Good. Very good.

Now if you want to, you can reach a deeper state of relaxation. . . .

Just imagine that your eyes are heavy, very heavy. . . . You find it impossible to open your eyes, no matter how hard you try. . . . They are so heavy . . . you are so relaxed . . . your eyes are shut tight . . . so heavy . . . you cannot open them.

You can stop trying to open them. Just let yourself go completely relaxed. Let yourself relax. At the count of three, you will notice that your eyes are locked tight . . . and you are completely relaxed. . . .

One . . . your eyes are heavy and heavier. . . .

Two . . . your lids are heavy . . . you are so tired. It will feel so good to close your eyes. . . . Your eyes are closing . . . you are feeling more relaxed. . . .

Three . . . shut your eyes, tight, tighter. Let your eyes roll up into the back of your head, just like you are looking up at your hair. . . .

Keep your eyes shut and breathe in . . . slowly, naturally. Deep breath. You are feeling more relaxed with every breath. If you wish to, you can go deeper into relaxation with every breath. . . .

Just listen to my voice. . . .

Just relax.

Suggestion

You can use this suggestion as part of your daily hypnosis practice session if you have a problem with excess weight gain.

You now feel completely relaxed and comfortable. Your stomach feels calm. Your mind is at peace. You feel perfectly at ease.

When you feel hungry, you crave fresh fruits and vegetables. You want to eat only those foods that you know will help to keep you and your baby healthy and strong. Your baby is growing inside you. Your baby needs healthful foods to grow. You are feeding your baby each time you eat something.

There is plenty of food for you and your baby. There is plenty of food for the next meal. Nothing to worry about. You have plenty of food when you need it.

You have permission to leave food on your plate if you feel full at mealtime. You want to choose healthful foods, but you do not want to eat more than your body needs. You are aware of everything you eat, and you do not want to eat too much of any food.

You drink skim milk rather than whole or two percent milk. You know the milk helps to nourish your baby and build your baby's bones and teeth. You drink water between meals, after meals, and during your meals if you remain thirsty after drinking your milk. You enjoy drinking cool, clean water. You can feel the water cleanse your body of any impurities. You can feel the water cleanse your baby.

You enjoy eating healthful foods. Your stomach feels satisfied and relaxed after eating. You feel calm, relaxed, and satisfied. Calm, relaxed, satisfied.

Closing

You can use the following script or one of the others described in Chapter 5.

In just a moment I will say the first four letters of the alphabet: A, B, C, and D. As I do so, you will begin to slowly open your eyes. Your eyes will be wide open when I reach letter D. You will feel relaxed and refreshed. You will look forward to the next hypnosis session when you will reach a deeper state of relaxation. You will feel as if you just awakened from a restful night of sleep.

Okay. Listen now. A . . . it's time to gradually open your eyes. Slowly now. You feel relaxed, at peace.

B . . . your eyes open a little more now. . . . The next time you enter hypnosis, you will find it easier to reach an even deeper state of relaxation. . . .

C . . . you are feeling a bit more alert. You will soon resume your normal state of awareness. You feel refreshed and alert and look forward to the joyful celebration of your baby's birth. . . . You will be able to relax and remain relaxed through every contraction.

D . . . open your eyes and feel wonderful.

7

▪ ▪ ▪ PUTTING TOGETHER YOUR BIRTHING TEAM
Finding the Help You Need

At one time, giving birth was essentially a one-woman show. Today, it usually involves a team of doctors, midwives, nurses, and other medical professionals. Although unexpected complications can arise, in most cases the event can go smoothly when Mom has the support of well-trained professionals who share her vision of the birth experience.

When it comes to using hypnosis as a form of anesthesia during delivery, discuss the matter with your obstetrician, midwife, or other medical professional well before your delivery. If your doctor supports your decision, your chances of successfully using hypnosis are much higher. "Most doctors will accept the use of hypnosis, but they usually aren't enthusiastic," says Marie Mongan. "Even after they see hypnosis used successfully, they tend to remain skeptical."

Few doctors have much experience using hypnosis as anesthesia, so you will need to assemble a birthing team that includes people who can support you in your efforts. You can practice hypnosis on your own using the techniques described in this book, but you will be most successful if your primary health-care provider is aware of and supportive of your desire to use hypnosis for pain management. If you want to work with a trained hypnotherapist, look for one with expertise in the use of hypnosis during pregnancy. If appropriate, you may also want to work with a midwife and a doula, a birth assistant who can comfort and nurture you throughout the delivery. In some cases, the midwife or doula has experience with hypnosis; in most cases, you will need to work with a separate hypnotherapist.

Finding a Hypnotist

Hypnotherapy is an unlicensed profession. In most states, anyone with a pocket watch and gold chain can claim to be a hypnotherapist without any special training or licensing. That means it's up to you to check into the qualifications of any hypnotherapist you may want to hire to assist with the delivery of your baby.

Before choosing a hypnotherapist, interview three or four prospective candidates. Be sure to ask about the person's experience using hypnosis during pregnancy. An expert therapist who is skilled at the use of hypnosis to help a person stop smoking or recover lost memories may not be the best one to help you with pain management during labor and delivery.

To find the right hypnotherapist, collect a list of prospective candidates, then take some time to interview them. First, obtain referrals from the American Society of Clinical Hypnosis and the Society for Clinical and Experimental Hypnosis. These two groups are the only nationally recognized organizations with a membership limited to licensed health-care professionals; members of these organizations must meet strict criteria for admission.

Don't be confused by the credentials issued by the dozens of organizations with official-sounding names, such as the American Board of Hypnotherapy, the American Council of Hypnotist Examiners, and the National Guild of Hypnotists, among others. These groups offer referrals and issue credentials, but they do not require that their members be medical professionals. Hypnotherapists can learn the art of hypnosis from professional societies, hypnosis institutes, individuals, or how-to books. Some of these postsecondary hypnosis training schools offer superior training, but others do not, and, unfortunately, it is difficult to differentiate between the two.

You may also want to contact the HypnoBirthing Institute, an organization dedicated to training hypnotherapists to assist during the birthing process. For a listing of how to contact these groups, see the resources section on pages 153–159. Also ask for referrals from physicians, friends, family members, coworkers, and the psychology departments of local universities.

Many hypnotherapists who specialize in childbirth offer both individual and group hypnosis sessions, or a combination of both. Group sessions are less expensive than individual sessions, but some people find them less effective. According to Nancy Barwick, a hypnobirthing therapist, groups should be limited to no more than three or four couples. It can be difficult to focus if more people are present.

Questions to Ask a Prospective Hypnotherapist

When interviewing hypnotherapists, you need to feel comfortable asking questions, even difficult questions. Most important, you need to trust your instincts and choose only someone who feels right to you. If you have any concerns about a person's qualifications, keep looking. Be sure to ask the following questions during the interview.

- *Are you a licensed medical professional?* Lay hypnotists are trained in hypnosis but lack medical, psychological, or other health-care training. A lay hypnotist may be certified as a hypnotist but not licensed as a medical professional. Professional credentials may be impressive, but you should not rely on them alone. A nonprofessional who is experienced in hypnotherapy may be better able to assist with your pregnancy than a well-schooled practitioner who lacks experience with the use of hypnosis during delivery. Being a medical professional should be a factor, but not the only factor, to look at when assessing a person's qualifications.

- *What kind of training have you had in hypnosis?* Look for someone who has had at least 150 hours of formal training in hypnosis; this applies to both professional and lay hypnotists.

- *Do you work full- or part-time with hypnosis?* The more someone practices hypnosis, the more competent he or she is apt to be.

- *What experience do you have working with pregnant women?* You want to choose someone with expertise in labor and delivery.

- *What are your fees? Does this cover only a fixed number of sessions? If so, how much would extra sessions cost?* Most hypnotherapists see women weekly for four to six weeks during pregnancy, but every practitioner has a different arrangement.

- *How many sessions do you anticipate that I will need to become proficient enough to use hypnosis during childbirth?* It is important that you have an understanding of the skills you will learn and the number of sessions it will take to learn them.

- *May I bring someone with me to the hypnosis sessions?* You probably want to include your spouse or birth assistant in the training so that this person can help provide hypnotic suggestions during labor.

- *May I tape-record the sessions?* Any hypnotherapist working with you on preparation for labor should encourage you to record the hypnotherapy sessions so that you can practice your skills on your own and reinforce the techniques taught during the session.

- *Of the pregnant women you have worked with, how many were successful in avoiding the use of pain medication during delivery?* Although some hypnotherapists may resist discussing their "success rate," you have a right to ask the question.

• *May I have the names and phone numbers of women you assisted in childbirth with hypnosis?* The most compelling referral is often a satisfied former patient.

• *Do you use hypnosis yourself?* A practitioner who believes in the technique will probably use it as well.

Questions to Ask Yourself When Choosing a Hypnotherapist

You must feel comfortable with your hypnotherapist in order for the technique to be successful during your pregnancy. You will need to feel relaxed and safe with any prospective therapist. After interviewing a candidate, ask yourself the following questions.

• Do I like the person?

• Do I trust him or her?

• Was I treated with respect?

• Did I like the sound of the person's voice? Was it annoying or distracting in any way?

• Did the person seem excited about my pregnancy?

- Did I feel comfortable enough with the person to allow myself to be passive?

- Did the therapist seem professional and competent?

- Was the person on time for our appointment?

- Did the person listen to me as an individual, or was I treated as just another pregnant woman?

Again, pay attention to your instincts. If a hypnotherapist doesn't feel right, keep searching until you find someone who does. You must feel comfortable with a hypnotist for the techniques to be most effective.

Finding a Midwife

The medical professional you choose to assist with your birth will play a vital role in determining what childbirth will be like for you. If you want a more natural birth experience, you can increase the odds by making sure your health-care provider supports anesthesia-free childbirth. Discuss the topic openly with your health-care provider very early in your pregnancy.

Though there are huge differences in philosophy and style, your basic choices include obstetricians, family practitioners, and certified nurse-midwives. Obstetricians handle most maternity care in the United States. They are medical doctors who have three or more years of specialty training in obstetrics and gynecology. Family practitioners are medical doctors who focus on the total health care of the individual and the family. They too have three years of training following medical school, including at least three months of obstetrics and gynecology.

Certified nurse-midwives specialize in the care of healthy women with low-risk pregnancies. They work with backup physicians who are on call to consult or take over in case of complications or emergency. The word *midwife* comes from the Old English word for "with women." This reflects the fact that certified nurse-midwives take a very supportive approach to labor and delivery. They tend to emphasize childbirth preparation and education and minimize the use of high-tech, invasive equipment. Some also have experience using hypnosis for pain control.

Midwives deliver babies in hospitals and birth centers and patients' homes. Certified nurse-midwives are registered nurses who have also completed a year or more of training at one of the nearly forty midwifery programs accredited by the American College of Nurse-Midwives. They have also passed board examinations issued by the ACNM.

Certified nurse-midwives provide first-class medical care. A study done by the U.S. Office of Technology Assessment determined that care provided by certified nurse-midwives is equivalent to a physician's care and that midwives often are better than physicians at providing services that require communication and preventive action. Also, reports by the National Institute of Medicine and the National Commission to Prevent Infant Mortality praise the contributions of certified nurse-midwives in reducing the incidence of low-birth-weight babies.

Certified nurse-midwives can practice in every state, but lay midwives cannot. Lay midwives aren't nurses; they have learned to deliver babies through self-study, apprenticeship, and experience. Some states license lay midwives and legally permit them to deliver babies; others consider their work the "illegal practice of medicine." If a lay midwife is not licensed, it is difficult to determine if she meets the necessary professional standards.

To verify the credentials of certified nurse-midwives, contact the American College of Nurse-Midwives listed in the resources section on page 157. To find out if a lay midwife is licensed in your state, contact the state board of medical examiners, usually located in the state capital.

Questions to Ask a Prospective Certified Nurse-Midwife

You should be diligent about interviewing prospective caregivers, but you should also follow your instincts. It's legitimate to make a decision based on a gut reaction, as long as you've done your best to ensure that the nurse-midwife you select is qualified and can provide the care you need.

- Do you have experience working with hypnosis as a form of anesthesia during labor and delivery?

- If not, would you be willing to work with a hypnotherapist?

- Are you a licensed, registered nurse? Where did you receive training?

- How many births have you attended? What complications have you witnessed and how were the problems handled?

- How often will we meet during pregnancy?

- At what stage of labor would you have me go to the hospital?

- What is your philosophy about the use of anesthesia and pain medication during labor?

- What is your fee?

- Do you participate with my insurance company or health-maintenance organization?

- May I have the names and phone numbers of women you have assisted in childbirth?

Questions to Ask Yourself About a Prospective Midwife

- Do I like the person?

- Do I feel confident in her abilities?

- Was I treated with respect?

- Did the person seem willing to act as my advocate throughout my pregnancy?

- Did the person seem excited about my pregnancy?

Finding a Doula

Even mothers need a little mothering, especially during childbirth. A doula (pronounced DOO la) is a woman who comforts and supports a woman during pregnancy and childbirth by offering both emotional and physical support. In fact, the word *doula* is a Greek word meaning "woman who serves."

A doula acts as a woman's advocate, offering words of encouragement, helping the mother stay focused and relaxed, and, for a woman using hypnosis, providing an environment that allows her to use hypnosis effectively for pain control. All too often, women who use anesthesia during delivery regret their choice, wishing that they had more encouragement to manage the pain naturally; a doula can provide support and help a woman withstand the temptation to say yes to drugs.

A number of studies have found advantages to delivering with a doula. According to a study published in the journal *Clinical Consultations in Obstetrics and Gynecology* in 1992, women working with a doula had 50 percent fewer caesarean deliveries and 40 percent fewer forceps deliveries, compared to women who did not work with doulas. They also had 25 percent shorter labors, and they were 60 percent less likely to use epidural anesthesia and 40 percent less apt to have needed artificial hormones to speed labor.

A doula does not make medical decisions; she is not trained as a doctor, nurse, or midwife. That is not to say she is uninformed; a doula should be well versed in the full range of medical options so that she can explain them to you and answer your questions, not so that she can make any medical recommendations. Some doulas have experience using hypnosis; all should be able to help you relax and practice the skills of self-hypnosis that you have learned in hypnotherapy.

The doula is called during labor and she stays with you until after the baby is born. She helps you cope with labor in any way that works. Because she is not a member of the immediate family, the doula is able to focus all of her energy on the mother and father.

As you might expect, doulas have been found to be most effective when they are known by the doctors and nurses at the hospital where you plan to deliver the baby. You will want to meet with a doula during the sixth or seventh month of your pregnancy, and at that time you might want to make sure that your doula introduces herself to the hospital staff if she has not already done so.

If you think your delivery would be enhanced by working with a doula, talk to your doctor about your intentions. Once you find a doula, write to the hospital and let the staff know that you plan to have a doula present at the delivery as an extra support person. Be sure to bring a copy of the letter of permission with you to the hospital to avoid conflict if a nurse tells you that hospital policy allows only family members to attend the birth.

Questions to Ask a Prospective Doula

- What professional training have you had?

- How long have you worked as a doula?

- How may births have you assisted?

- At which hospitals have you assisted with deliveries?

- At what point in labor do you want to be called?

- Do you do internal exams? What medical tasks can you do?

- Do you offer assistance with breast-feeding?

- How many children do you have? What were your birth experiences like?

- What specific services do you provide as a doula?

- Do you have experience working with hypnosis?

- What doctors have you worked with?

- Who will assist us if you are not available at the time of our baby's birth?

- What is your fee? Is part of the fee refundable if you do not attend the birth?

- May we have client references?

Questions to Ask Yourself About a Prospective Doula

- Do you feel comfortable with the person?

- Does the doula share your philosophy about childbirth?

- Is this a person your spouse feels he can work with?

- Does the doula have experience working with hypnosis?

- Is the doula willing to learn more about hypnosis if she doesn't know much about it?

- Will the doula be available to attend your birth?

You should interview two or three prospective doulas before choosing one; after all, the person you choose will be with you during one of the most important experiences of your life.

For more information on doulas or to obtain a referral to

a qualified professional in your area, contact the Association of Labor Assistants and Childbirth Educators or Doulas of North America. (For more information, see the resources listed on page 159.)

8

■ ■ ■ QUESTIONS AND ANSWERS ABOUT HYPNOSIS

Hypnosis doesn't get the respect it deserves. On television and in the movies, hypnotists are usually portrayed as either Svengali-like masters who exert absolute control over their subjects or as goofy entertainers who lure audience members onto the stage and then make their prey perform humiliating (but amusing) acts.

As you know from reading this far, hypnosis is a serious tool, which can be used to help you experience a more enjoyable, natural labor and delivery. Still, you may have some questions about hypnosis and how it works. The following questions may help clear up some of your misconceptions.

Are there any people who should avoid hypnosis?
Hypnosis for pain control is considered safe for all pregnant women. As mentioned earlier, the technique can be used by almost anyone who has an understanding of the language being spoken.

Hypnosis can also be used by psychologists and psychiatrists as a tool to explore painful childhood memories. In such

situations, the technique should be used only by a professional.

*Aside from pain relief, are there other benefits to using hypnosis
during delivery?*
Yes. According to a study published in 1990 in the *Journal of
Consulting and Clinical Psychology,* researchers at the University of Wisconsin studied two groups of women in their ninth
month of pregnancy. The women in both groups were of
similar age, health, and psychological makeup. As part of the
study, all of the women attended six childbirth classes offered
by their obstetricians, which included relaxation and
breathing exercises. Half of the women received training in
hypnosis as well. The women who were trained in hypnosis
had shorter labors, used less medication, and experienced less
pain during delivery, and their babies had higher Apgar scores
(a measure of a baby's overall health in the moments after
birth). In addition, the women who used hypnosis experienced less depression after delivery. They achieved these impressive benefits by reducing their awareness of pain. They
were able to approach delivery with a relaxed body, which
allowed the birthing muscles to work in harmony and without resistance from tensed muscles elsewhere in the body.

*Can a person be made to do things against her will while in a
hypnotic trance?*
No. No one can be forced to do anything against her will or
in opposition to her personal value system while in a hypnotic
trance. Many people feel nervous about losing control or sur-

rendering their will while under hypnosis, but this is not possible. Remember, a person remains fully aware of everything that happens while under hypnosis. A hypnotic subject remains in complete control throughout a session of hypnosis, and a hypnotic suggestion works only if a person chooses to accept it.

When people participate in stage acts and behave in foolish ways for entertainment, it sometimes appears that they are being dominated or controlled by the hypnotist, but this is not true. Stage hypnotists choose volunteers who are cooperative and enjoy the attention of "performing" in a show. These entertainers have an ability to focus on good subjects, which creates the impression that these people are under the control of the hypnotist. At any time, any person in such a situation has the power to stop the show and return to his or her seat. The person is acting voluntarily at all times.

Can a person be hypnotized against her will?
Again, no. Although it is true that almost anyone can be hypnotized, he or she must be a willing participant. A subject does have the power to resist hypnotic suggestions. A hypnotherapist does not impose a hypnotic trance on a subject; instead, the subject chooses to enter the hypnotic trance, as guided by the therapist.

Will a person remember what happens during a hypnosis session?
Most people remember everything that happens during hypnosis. A small percentage of people—typically those who can enter the deepest levels of hypnotic trance—may experience

hypnotic amnesia, but this is usually at the suggestion of the hypnotherapist. When using hypnosis in childbirth, there is no reason to induce amnesia.

Does a person have to go into a deep trance to experience anesthesia?
Fortunately, no. Pain control and anesthesia can be induced in a medium-depth hypnotic trance. A person does not need to have any special skills or a particular hypnotic ability to be able to benefit from hypnotic anesthesia.

If asked, will a person reveal personal secrets while in a hypnotic trance?
No, your secrets are safe. Again, the subject is able to control her behavior while hypnotized. A person can even lie while in a trance, which is why testimony given while under hypnosis is not admissible in a court of law. When using hypnosis for anesthesia during childbirth, there is no reason for a partner or hypnotherapist to ask any questions that should make a person feel vulnerable. If such questions were asked, the subject's subconscious mind would probably ignore the questions or pull the person out of the trance.

How does a person know she has been hypnotized?
Many times people come out of a trance and find it difficult to believe that they have been hypnotized. There are, however, a number of indications that a person has been in a trance. First, a person will feel a profound sense of relaxation throughout her entire body. Any fatigue or tension that was present before the session usually disappears during hypnosis.

Typically, a person's eyelids feel heavy when the hypnotist suggests they feel that way. As the state of hypnosis deepens, the person may feel unable to open her eyes, but this doesn't matter because her attention is focused on the hypnotist's words and suggestions. As the session continues, the person's attention filters out all outside noises and distractions, paying attention only to the sound of the hypnotist's words.

During the state of hypnosis, the mind develops an almost single-minded purpose—to follow the suggestion of the hypnotist. In this state, a person can use her mind to control pain and to introduce other behavioral changes in the subconscious mind.

At the end of a hypnotic session, most people "awaken" feeling rested, refreshed, and almost euphoric. In addition, many report a distortion in the perception of time. Some people assume that a few minutes have passed when it has really been much longer; others feel that they were hypnotized for hours when they were actually in a trance for only a few minutes. Often this perception of time can be affected by a hypnotic suggestion while the subject is in a trance. For example, sometimes hypnotherapists give women the suggestion that the passing of ten minutes will feel like one minute; in this way a woman can hurry along her labor by changing her perception of time.

Does a person have to stare at a swinging pocket watch to enter a hypnotic trance?
Not necessarily. The pocket watch cliché was started because a monotonous swinging motion gives a person something to focus on and the repetitive motion rapidly lulls the person

into a state of profound relaxation. In many cases a person is asked to stare at something or to close her eyes and visualize something in order to introduce a hypnotic trance.

Is hypnosis covered by insurance?
It depends on your insurance company, but a growing number of policies cover hypnosis. In fact, in 1996 a panel convened by the National Institutes of Health recommended that insurance companies reimburse patients for the cost of hypnosis used for pain control. Currently, many health-maintenance organizations pay for hypnotherapy if it is used with the approval of your primary-care physician.

Can most women who use hypnosis avoid the use of all anesthesia during childbirth?
Most people are capable of achieving hypnotic anesthesia, if they are willing and able to work at it. However, many women go into labor early or fail to practice on a regular basis. As a result, experts estimate that about half of the women who undergo hypnotic training actually deliver without any chemical anesthesia. It must be noted, however, that the amount of anesthesia used by women who use hypnosis tends to be significantly less than the average amount used by women without training in hypnosis. In addition, some women use hypnosis during childbirth to promote relaxation and minimize anxiety rather than as a substitute for chemical anesthesia.

What happens to a woman if her partner or hypnotherapist is forced to leave before bringing her out of the hypnotic trance?

The patient wouldn't be stuck in a trance if the hypnotist left before formally closing the session. The person would either fall into a deep sleep and then awaken naturally, or she would come out of the trance immediately. Keep in mind that the hypnotic relationship requires give and take between the hypnotist and the subject. If the hypnotist leaves, the lines of communication close down.

Is it possible for a person to be "a little bit" hypnotized?
It's impossible to be "a little bit" pregnant, but a person can be "a little bit" hypnotized. As noted earlier, there are several different depths of hypnosis. A person does not need to enter the deepest states of hypnosis to be able to control pain. With practice, most people can train themselves to increase their depth of hypnosis, if they wish to do so.

Does the mind work differently while in a hypnotic trance?
Yes, it tends to process information very literally. Sometimes hypnotists demonstrate this fact by asking a person in a hypnotic trance to raise her hand. In a state of normal consciousness, most people will raise their entire arm. When in a hypnotic trance, a person will raise only the hand, from the wrist to the fingertips. Because the mind processes language very precisely while under hypnosis, it is important for a hypnotist to carefully choose the exact language when preparing a hypnotic script.

How does the body respond when the mind is in a hypnotic trance?
In most cases, when a person enters a hypnotic trance she is

instructed to relax and become calm and centered. In this state of relaxation, a person's blood pressure drops, breathing and heart rate slow, and her muscles relax. Often a person's mouth falls open and her eyelids flutter. Sometimes tears stream down a person's cheeks, not as an emotional response to anything she is experiencing but because the tear ducts relax during hypnosis.

Should a person seek the assistance of a professional hypnotherapist?
Most women can benefit from working with a skilled hypnotherapist who has expertise in assisting pregnant women. Choose a hypnotist with care; an excellent hypnotist is able to customize his or her approach to match an individual's personality, vocabulary, and areas of interest. Ideally, a hypnotic script should reflect the subject's speech patterns and experiences. The better the words reflect a person's individual situation, the more likely the hypnotic suggestions will be effective and long-lasting.

How much does hypnosis usually cost?
Most hypnotherapists charge $200 to $400 for a series of sessions on hypnosis and childbirth, including several individual sessions and several group sessions. Additional private sessions usually cost $50 to $100 or so, but prices vary widely by geographic region and by the training of the hypnotherapist. Be sure to talk with the hypnotherapist about the cost of the session and the number of sessions that might be required before making a commitment to work with someone.

Will the hypnotherapist attend the birth?
It depends on the arrangements you make with the hypnotherapist. "The success of hypnosis does not depend on a birth assistant being there," says Marie Mongan. You need to practice on your own, so you should not assume that the technique will work only if the hypnotherapist is present. In some cases, hypnotherapists attend a birth at a mother's request, but arrangements should be worked out well in advance.

What is the difference between hypnosis and the Dick-Read method of natural childbirth?
Hypnosis and the Dick-Read method share a number of similarities. The Dick-Read method, an approach to childbirth education developed by Dr. Grantly Dick-Read, a British physician, and published in his book *Natural Childbirth* in 1933, emphasizes that childbirth should be a satisfying experience and that a woman need have no more pain in childbirth than she is willing to accept. Dr. Dick-Read believed that women should be educated about the biological and psychological changes in childbirth; he believed pain could be controlled through an awareness of the emotions a woman experiences during labor. The Dick-Read method argues that a doctor's suggestion can raise a patient's pain threshold and reduce her need for anesthesia. However, the Dick-Read method differs from hypnosis most dramatically in how the techniques use the mind. Specifically, the Dick-Read method deals only with conscious fear and tension, whereas hypnosis works with the subconscious as well.

Can hypnosis help me if I have a caesarean delivery?
Yes, hypnosis can help you relax and accept your doctor's

decision to deliver your baby surgically. The technique can be used to focus your mental and emotional energy on having a healthy baby, rather than having a particular type of childbirth experience. In addition, hypnosis can be very helpful in speeding recovery after a C-section.

9

WHEN THINGS DON'T GO AS PLANNED
If Anesthesia Is Necessary

Sarah Duncan had every intention of using anesthesia during the delivery of her second child. Still, she wanted to use hypnosis to overcome the fear of childbirth she had after the traumatic forceps delivery of her first child after a sixteen-hour labor. "My goal was not to avoid all drugs," said thirty-one-year-old Sarah. "I wanted help with anxiety so that I could have a more serene childbirth experience." Sarah described the birth of nine-pound Maxwell as "fabulous." "Hypnosis allowed me to have the kind of birth I wanted—short, easy, and peaceful."

Although Sarah planned on using pain-relieving drugs during her labor, some women use hypnosis to avoid the use of anesthesia. Despite their intentions, many women find it very difficult to resist pain-relieving drugs when they are offered. Hypnosis helps them get through the early stages of labor, but they feel tempted to use medication if they break their concentration or if they are repeatedly offered anesthesia. Too often women accept drugs, only to regret the decision after the baby is born. "I wish I could have held out longer," is a common refrain.

Often a spouse unwittingly encourages a woman to use anesthesia because he finds it almost unbearable to see his beloved partner in pain. Many doctors and nurses likewise push drugs on their patients. Midwives can be helpful in supporting a woman who does not wish to use medication.

Of course, medication may be necessary when a labor is prolonged, stuck, or induced, but under normal circumstances it is important to respect and support the mother's desire to rely on hypnosis—mind over labor—to control discomfort. Rather than offering a woman drugs, her partner should offer support and encouragement.

Well-meaning friends and family members often question a woman's choice of using hypnosis for pain control during childbirth. They may ask, "When you have a severe headache, do you refuse to take an aspirin?" Or "Would you have a root canal without being numbed?" The difference, of course, is that during headaches and dental procedures, there is no risk to an unborn child. And, unlike childbirth, a visit to the dentist is not a significant social or psychological transition. Dental work is required when something in the body has gone wrong and needs to be repaired; childbirth is a natural process that does not automatically need to be treated as a medical problem. In keeping with the dental analogy, anesthesia is not required when baby teeth fall out (a natural process). Likewise, women's bodies are designed to give birth, and they do not necessarily require anesthesia to do so.

It is important to note that the body prepares for discomfort during labor and delivery by releasing the natural chemical painkillers known as endorphins. When a woman uses analgesics and anesthetics, she is sending a message to her brain that the pain has passed and the endorphins are no longer required. As a result, when the chemical painkillers wear off, many women experience a rebound effect of increased pain because their bodies are less equipped to handle it. Once a woman begins to use painkilling drugs, it is often very difficult to stop using them until the delivery is complete. This does not occur after hypnosis.

Painkilling Drugs

The practice of using painkilling treatments to control discomfort during childbirth was not widespread before the nineteenth century. That changed in 1847, when a physician named James Simpson first administered chloroform to a woman who was overwrought with anxiety and fear of childbirth because she had previously given birth to a stillborn child after a three-day labor. The drug left the woman unconscious during the delivery; when she awoke, she had not experienced any pain. In fact, the doctor had a difficult time convincing her that labor was over and that the baby she was holding was actually her own. Dr. Simpson was so delighted with the results that he began using chloroform in every labor he attended.

The practice caught on, and over the years doctors experimented with different sedatives. "Twilight sleep" was the most popular form of anesthesia in the United State for nearly half a century. This soothing-sounding treatment consisted of an injection of a combination of morphine and Scopolamine. The potent painkiller was devised in Germany in the early twentieth century and used as late as 1980 in some hospitals. When treated, a woman didn't feel or remember anything about her labor.

Most doctors assumed that the practice presented no harm to the infants, though we now know that this was not the case. Ironically, it was when doctors began to use electronic fetal monitors that they saw the effects of "twilight sleep" on the baby and finally stopped using the drug cocktail. Over the years, this combination has been replaced with narcotics and epidural anesthesia.

We have known since the 1960s that all obstetric medications given to the mother cross the placenta and affect the baby. This applies to all medications, whether they are given to induce labor, to relieve pain, or to anesthetize. Contrary to what many women are told, this includes the regional anesthetics used in epidurals. These drugs enter the baby's bloodstream; some studies have found that the anesthetic levels in the baby's blood can be as high as one-third of the mother's blood levels. It takes about forty-eight hours for a newborn to remove the epidural anesthetic from its system.

What does this medication do to the baby? Researchers have found that babies born to mothers who had epidural anesthesia tend to demonstrate more trembling, irritability, and immature motor activity on the first day, compared to babies born to mothers who did not take medication. It was not until the fifth day that the two groups of babies exhibited similar behavior. Babies born to mothers who used the labor-inducing drug Pitocin along with the epidural showed an even greater depression of motor activity than those babies whose mothers used an epidural alone.

Of course, it is important also to bear in mind that in

instances of real need, the judicial and minimal use of medication is usually beneficial. However, mothers are rarely well informed about the hazards or side effects involved in taking such medications and are deluded into assuming that there are no risks.

Narcotics

Used to take the edge off pain, narcotics are usually given as intramuscular injections. Some women find that they make labor more tolerable; others feel that the drugs cause them to feel as if they are losing control.

These drugs have possible side effects on the mother, such as nausea and dizziness, and they slow the mother's breathing and respiration, somewhat reducing the baby's oxygen supply. To reduce the mother's nausea, narcotics are often mixed with sedatives, and these too enter the baby's bloodstream and cause sleepiness.

It is now common knowledge that Demerol and similar drugs can depress the baby's respiratory system and jeopardize the start of breathing after birth. Although anesthesiologists try to prevent breathing problems by timing the dosage of the drug to wear off sufficiently before birth, some babies must be resuscitated to start breathing after birth.

Traces of these medications typically remain in the baby's circulatory system after birth, so that in addition to adjusting to life outside the womb, the baby's system has the added burden of detoxification. In some cases, they can depress the baby's sucking reflex, which can hinder breast-feeding.

Epidural Anesthesia

This is the common name for the injection of a regional anesthetic into the epidural space between two lumbar vertebrae in the lower spine. The result is a blocking of pain impulses, causing numbness from the waist to the thighs or down to the toes.

Even though the drugs used for epidurals do not affect the body as Demerol does, we know that they enter the baby's circulation and brain tissue within minutes. Their immediate and long-term effects on the baby's neurological development are relatively unknown, despite the widespread use of this form of pain relief.

The mother can experience side effects, most commonly a severe headache if the membrane surrounding the spinal cord is accidentally penetrated by the needle during the injection.

In addition, epidural anesthesia increases the chances that obstetric intervention will be required.

- Contractions tend to be less efficient after epidural anesthesia. For one thing, the woman is required to lie down flat, which makes labor less efficient. In most cases, a woman who has an epidural must be hooked up to an epidural pump, an intravenous line, and a fetal monitor.

- Epidural anesthesia minimizes the release of oxytocin, the body's natural labor-inducing chemical. The sensations a woman feels when the cervix is dilating signal the brain to release more oxytocin, a natural chemical that stimulates labor and speeds cervical dilation. An epidural diminishes or deadens those sensations, which short-circuits this feedback system and slows labor. (Hypnosis does not slow labor; it hastens it by allowing the uterine muscles to work with minimal resistance. The natural chemicals are released, but the brain does not interpret the messages as pain.)

- Epidural anesthesia lowers levels of endorphins (the body's natural painkillers), which further slows labor. Endorphin levels correlate with the release of oxytocin.

- Epidural anesthesia can also lower the mother's blood pressure, which can decrease the oxygen circulation to the baby and slow the baby's heart rate. To prevent complications, most doctors require that a woman have continuous electronic fetal monitoring if she has an epidural. In addition, many women receive intravenous fluids to maintain an appropriate blood pressure. This can, in turn, cause swelling in the woman's feet, legs, and breasts. As you might imagine, these procedures all add to the stress associated with childbirth.

- With epidural anesthesia, a woman can no longer feel the natural sensations that tell her when to shift positions to stimulate labor. Normally, a woman's body sends her messages of how to move to make labor most productive. A woman with an epidural cannot receive such messages, nor is she able to act on them because she cannot move freely.

- Epidural anesthesia increases the chances a baby will need to be pulled out with a vacuum extractor (suction) or with forceps. The epidural anesthesia can weaken a woman's urge to push when she is fully dilated and ready to deliver her baby. Normally, when the cervix is dilated, the baby's head slips farther down into the pelvis, stretching the muscles in the pelvic floor. This pressure triggers a desire within the woman to push the baby out. If these pelvic nerves have been anesthetized, a woman is five times more likely to need assistance with the pushing phase.

- The pushing phase of labor tends to be longer in women who have had epidural anesthesia. One study in 1981 found that women with an epidural took an average of 100 minutes to push the baby out and women with an epidural and Pitocin took 84 minutes, compared with 47 minutes in an unmedicated mother.

- A woman is more likely to receive labor-enhancing drugs if she has epidural anesthesia. Because the contractions can become less efficient, in many cases labor is much longer and a doctor may recommend that the contractions be artificially stimulated with an oyxtocic (Pitocin) drip.

- Epidural anesthesia increases the likelihood that a woman will require catheterization. Because the anesthesia numbs the bladder, a woman is unable to respond to her body's signals that she needs to urinate. In some cases a doctor prescribes the use of a urinary catheter until the epidural wears off in several hours. Catheterization brings an added risk of bladder infection and problems with urinary incontinence. Studies show that there is a 700 percent increase in urinary incontinence three months after a woman receives catheritization with an epidural. Even a year later, incontinence remains 200 percent higher than in mothers who did not have epidural anesthesia.

- Women who have epidural anesthesia are three times more likely than women who give birth naturally to have deep vaginal tears extending into the rectum. In addition to being painful, these deep tears can cause fecal incontinence and chronic pain during sexual intercourse.

- Women who receive epidural anesthesia sometimes develop a complication known as "epidural fever." Within two or three hours after an epidural is started, many women experience an increase in temperature of about 0.1 degree per hour. An estimated one out of every four women who receive an epidural develops a fever within four hours, and almost half experience an increase in temperature within eight hours. This fever can cause a dramatic increase in the baby's heart rate. Women who develop a fever may require intravenous antibiotic treatment, as well as interventions to speed labor, such as Pitocin, forceps or vacuum extraction, or caesarean delivery.

- A woman is more likely to require a caesarean delivery if she has epidural anesthesia. The increased monitoring and immobilization can cause a cascading effect of complications that ultimately result in surgical delivery. Studies have shown that using continuous fetal monitoring increases the caesarean rate by two to three times. One study found a caesarean rate of 17 percent among women who had epidural anesthesia and only 2 percent in women who did not have anesthesia, even though both groups of women were considered essentially equivalent. Studies have also found that the earlier epidural anesthesia is started, the more likely a woman is to have a caesarean delivery. Researchers found a 50 percent increase in caesarean birth rate when the epidural was started when the woman's cervix was two centimeters dilated, a 33 percent increase when the woman was three centimeters dilated, and a 26 percent increase when she was four centimeters dilated.

When Medical Intervention Is Required

No matter how much you practice your hypnosis and how well you plan for the birth of your child, your birth experience may not go according to plan. When the unexpected happens, be ready to let go of your attachment to a certain type of experience so that you can do whatever is necessary to ensure the safe delivery of your healthy baby. In some cases, medications may be necessary, either to alter the course of labor or to help manage pain, and *this is okay*.

The two most common situations requiring medical intervention are when labor fails to progress and when a woman has her labor induced by her physician. In some cases, hypnosis may be all a woman requires to manage the discomfort of these medical interventions, but in other situations chemical anesthesia may also be required. Again, it is important to stress that your goal—and your hypnotic suggestions—should focus on a safe birth experience.

Failure to Progress

In some cases, a woman experiences strong, regular contractions for more than four hours, but her cervix fails to dilate beyond a certain point. Normal labor can follow a number of patterns—some women have strong, fast labors while other progress slowly but steadily. Labor is considered normal when, after reaching four centimeters, dilation progresses at least one centimeter every hour or two. To stimulate contractions and jump-start labor, a woman can try walking, massage, nipple stimulation, and other techniques recommended by her caretakers.

If there is no change in dilation after two hours of good labor, a doctor may recommend medical intervention, such as the use of the contraction-enhancing drug Pitocin. Pitocin is synthetic oxytocin that works by stimulating the smooth muscles of the uterus and blood vessels; it makes uterine contractions stronger and more frequent.

Pitocin-enhanced contractions can cause additional discomfort. Some women receiving Pitocin can remain relaxed using only hypnosis, but others request pain medication at this point. In such cases, use of epidural anesthesia may actually normalize labor and prevent unnecessary birth trauma. The prolonged stress of unproductive labor exhausts the mother physically and emotionally and raises her adrenaline levels. This excess adrenaline actually neutralizes the oxytocin and weakens the contractions and slows cervical dilation. Once a woman reaches this point, the anesthesia can be helpful in allowing her to rest and give her body a chance to prepare for the baby's delivery.

Pitocin Induction

To protect the health of the mother or child, physicians sometimes recommend that a woman have her labor induced rather than wait for labor to occur naturally. In most cases, the labor is artificially brought on with the drug Pitocin, which is also used when labor does not progress (see previous section). Induction is common among overdue mothers who have not given birth at forty-two weeks' gestation. Pitocin is also used when a woman's water has broken but her contractions are weak or haven't started after twelve hours or so.

Although hypnosis can be used to control Pitocin-induced labor, some women find it more difficult to do so because the contractions tend to come on quickly. In addition, Pitocin-induced contractions tend to be more frequent and intense than natural contractions. In addition, a cervix that is "unripe" (long, thick, firm, closed, or little dilated) when labor is induced is likely to dilate slowly. Since Pitocin is administered through an intravenous line, a woman must be confined to a bed and tethered to monitoring equipment.

When labor is induced, a woman is more likely to use epidural anesthesia. In some cases, this is appropriate because, as with the failure to progress described above, anesthesia may be needed to lower adrenaline levels and allow the mother to relax and the contractions to resume.

■ ■ ■

Even though hypnosis can be used as anesthesia to control discomfort when Pitocin or other drugs are administered, it is almost never used in situations when a woman requires a caesarean delivery. Hypnosis can keep a woman calm before the procedure and can speed recovery afterward, but few women would want to rely on it exclusively during major surgery.

It is important to understand the medical interventions that may be required during childbirth and to appreciate that there are times that medicinal anesthesia is necessary or desirable. Do your best to use the power of hypnosis—the power of your mind—to imagine the type of birth experience you want. However, it is essential that you never lose sight of your ultimate goal—a safe delivery for you and your baby.

In many ways, hypnosis is something of a miracle. Using the power of your subconscious mind, you can alter the course of your labor and short-circuit the pain receptors in your brain. This is an impressive example of the miracle of the mind, but more impressive still is the miracle of birth itself.

RECOMMENDED READING

Arms, Suzanne. *Immaculate Deception II: Myth, Magic & Birth.* Berkeley: Celestial Arts, 1996.

Austin, Valerie. *Self Hypnosis: A Safe Self-Help Guide.* San Francisco: Thorsons, 1994.

Balaskas, Janet. *Active Birth: The New Approach to Giving Birth Naturally.* Boston: Harvard Common Press, 1992.

Caprio, Frank, M.D., and Joseph R. Berger. *Healing Yourself with Self-Hypnosis.* New York: Prentice Hall Press, 1998.

Crabtree, A. *From Mesmer to Freud: Magnetic Sleep and the Roots of Psychological Healing.* New Haven: Yale University Press, 1993.

England, Pam, CNM, MA, and Rob Horowitz, Ph.D. *Birthing from Within.* Albuquerque: Partera Press, 1998.

Hewitt, William W. *Hypnosis: A Power Program for Self-Improvement, Changing Your Life and Helping Others.* St. Paul, MN: Llewellyn Publications, 1996.

———. *Hypnosis for Beginners: Reach New Levels of Awareness and Achievement.* St. Paul, MN: Llewellyn Publications, 1997.

Hunter, C. Roy, M. S. *Master the Power of Self-Hypnosis*. New York: Sterling Publishing, 1998.

Jones, Carl. *Mind Over Labor: A Breakthrough Guide to Giving Birth*. New York: Penguin, 1987.

Klaus, Marshall H., M.D., John H. Kennell, M.D., and Phyllis H. Klaus, M.Ed., CSW. *Mothering the Mother: How a Doula Can Help You Have a Shorter, Easier, and Healthier Birth*. Reading, MA: Perseus Books, 1993.

Kroger, William, M.D. *Childbirth with Hypnosis*. North Hollywood, CA: Wilshire Book Company, 1961.

Lieberman, Adrienne B. *Easing Labor Pain: The Complete Guide to a More Comfortable and Rewarding Birth*. Boston: Harvard Common Press, 1992.

McCutcheon, Susan. *Natural Childbirth the Bradley Way*. New York: Penguin, 1996.

O'Neill, Michelle Leclaire, Ph.D., R. N. *Creative Childbirth: How You Can Easily Give Birth in Comfort and Without Fear Through the Leclaire Method*. Los Angeles: Papyrus, 1993.

Peterson, Gayle, Ph.D. *An Easier Childbirth: A Mother's Guide for Birthing Normally*. Berkeley: Shadow & Light Publications, 1993.

Temes, Roberta, Ph.D. *The Complete Idiot's Guide to Hypnosis*. Indianapolis: Alpha Books, 2000.

ORGANIZATIONS

Hypnosis and Visualization

American Board of Hypnotherapy
16842 Von Karman Avenue
Suite 475
Irvine, CA 92606
(800) 872-9996
www.hypnosis.com

The ABH offers free referrals to its 10,000 members, who have completed training from an approved school and been certified and registered; membership requires annual training updates.

American Council of Hypnotist Examiners
700 S. Central Avenue
Glendale, CA 91204
(818) 242-1159
(800) 894-9766
www.sonic.net/hypno/ache.html

The council is a nonprofit professional organization that aims to self-regulate hypnotherapists. Regional examining boards handle examinations and certification. The council provides referrals to more than 18,000 qualified members.

American Music Therapy Association
8455 Colesville Road
Suite 1000
Silver Spring, MD 20910
(301) 589-3300
www.musictherapy.org

The association provides information on the benefits of music therapy and relaxation. The group offers referrals to people who use music as part of their relaxation exercises.

American Society of Clinical Hypnosis
33 West Grand Avenue
Suite 402
Chicago, IL 60610
(312) 645-9810
www.asch.net

The society provides general information on hypnosis and gives referrals to its qualified professionals.

Biofeedback Certification Institute of America
10200 West 44th Avenue
Suite 304
Wheat Ridge, CO 80033

(303) 420-2902
www.bcia.org

The institute offers free referrals to more than 1,500 practitioners who are trained and certified in various types of biofeedback therapy. For a list of practitioners, send a stamped, self-addressed business-size envelope.

Center for Mind-Body Medicine
5225 Connecticut Avenue, NW
Suite 414
Washington, DC 20015
(202) 966-7338
www.cmbm.org

The center provides information on the use of mind-body techniques to control pain and promote healing.

National Board for Certified Clinical Hypnotherapists, Inc.
8750 Georgia Avenue
Suite 142-E
Silver Spring, MD 20901
(301) 608-0123
(800) 449-8144
www.natboard.com

NBCCH was organized in 1991 as an educational, scientific, and professional organization dedicated to professionalizing the practice of hypnotherapy. The board offers certification of hypnotists who meet specific eligibility requirements.

National Guild of Hypnotists
P.O. Box 308
Merrimack, NH 03054
(603) 429-9438
www.ngh.net

The guild provides general information on hypnotherapy, as well as referrals to certified hypnotherapists.

Society for Clinical and Experimental Hypnosis
2201 Hadder Road
Suite 1
Pullman, WA 99163
(509) 332-7555
http://sunsite.utk.edu/ijceh

The society provides referrals to qualified professionals; it also offers general information on hypnosis.

World Hypnosis Organization, Inc.
2521 W. Montrose Avenue
Chicago, IL 60618
(847) 455-3792
www.worldhypnosis.org

This is a nonprofit educational organization dedicated to professional, charitable, scientific, and educational research on hypnosis.

Childbirth and Childbirth Classes

American Academy of Husband-Coached Childbirth
(the Bradley Method)

P.O. Box 5224
Sherman Oaks, CA 91413-5224
(800) 423-2397
(818) 788-6662
www.naturalbirth.org

The organization provides information on the Bradley method of natural childbirth and offers a directory of qualified teachers.

American College of Nurse-Midwives
818 Connecticut Avenue, NW
Suite 900
Washington, DC 20006
(202) 728-9860
(888) 643-9433 for referral service
www.midwife.org

The organization provides general information on midwifery as well as a referral service to qualified midwives.

International Association of Parents and Professionals for Safe Alternatives in Childbirth (NAPSAC, International)
Route 4, Box 646
Marble Hill, MO 63764
(573) 238-2010

An umbrella organization for the alternative birth movement, NAPSAC offers a quarterly newsletter, a mail-order book service, and an international directory of alternative birth services.

International Childbirth Education Association
P.O. Box 20048
Minneapolis, MN 55420-0048
(612) 854-8660
www.icea.org

ICEA offers an interdisciplinary approach to birth education. Members remain autonomous, creating their own policies and programs. ICEA member groups offer classes, a journal, and a catalog of books and pamphlets on childbirth and family-centered maternity care.

Lamaze International
1200 19th Street, NW
Suite 300
Washington, DC 20036
(800) 368-4404
www.lamaze-childbirth.com

The oldest childbirth education program in America, ASPO/Lamaze provides referrals to local certified Lamaze instructors. Videos, books, and pamphlets on pregnancy and labor are also available by mail order.

Midwives Alliance of North America
P.O. Box 175
Newton, KS 67114
(316) 283-4543
www.mana.org

The alliance holds regional and national conferences, publishes a newsletter, and aims to build cooperation among midwives to promote midwifery as a standard of health care. MANA can provide you with information on midwifery and referrals to midwives in your area.

Doulas

Association of Labor Assistants and Childbirth Educators
P.O. Box 382724
Cambridge, MA 02238
(617) 441-2500
http://server4.hypermart.net/alacehq

The association provides general information on doulas and labor assistants; it also offers referrals to qualified professionals.

Doulas of North America
13513 North Grove Drive
Alpine, UT 84004
(801) 756-7331
www.dona.com

The group offers general information on the use of doulas during pregnancy; it also offers referrals to qualified professionals.

WEB SITES

You can find a wealth of information about hypnosis—as well as other pregnancy-related topics—on the Internet. The Web sites for the national organizations on hypnosis are included with the listings of the organizations in the preceding section. The following Web sites cover hypnosis as a general topic or offer links to other relevant sites.

http://health.yahoo.com/health/Alternative_Medicine/
Alternative_Therapies/Hypnotherapy/
   This site provides general information on hypnosis, as well as links to related Web sites and chat rooms.

www.childbirth.org
   This searchable database offers information on a range of pregnancy-related topics.

www.hypnosis.com
   This comprehensive site offers listings of books, resources, conferences, and educational facilities that deal with hyp-

nosis. It provides general information on hypnosis as well as an extensive listing of links to related Web sites.

www.hypno-analysis.org

This is the Web site for the International Association of Hypnoanalysists. The site includes frequently asked questions, links to related sites, and a searchable database of member practitioners nationwide.

www.hypnobirthing.com

This is the Web site of HypnoBirthing Childbirth Education, a copyrighted childbirth education method. The site includes referrals to birth assistants trained in this method.

INDEX